Health Reforms in Post-Communist Eastern Europe

"Tamara Popic's excellent book significantly advances our understanding of the different reform trajectories of public health care systems in Eastern European countries after the end of the communist regime. Her book particularly focuses on reforms that aimed at marketizing health care systems in three exemplary cases, Slovenia, Poland, and the Czech Republic. Rather than merely assessing how partisan politics, institutions, and professional interests affected such reform trajectories, Popic's study is based on a novel and original argument emphasizing the importance of endogenous factors, such as policy learning and policymakers' prior exposure to experiences with market mechanisms, in shaping policy change. This innovative argument is supported by masterfully crafted in-depth case studies based on a wealth of original sources such as expert interviews, legal documents, and parliamentary debates. Overall, Popic's book is a substantive and timely addition to an understudied dimension of the restructuring process of post-communist welfare state: the field of public health care."

—Evelyne Hübscher, *Central European University, Austria*

"After the fall of communism, healthcare marketization invested Eastern European countries, often to the detriment of equality and fairness. The volume reveals, however, that in the last three decades such wave of reforms generated a variety of marketized healthcare arrangements across countries. Then, carefully investigating the "politics of health privatization" in Slovenia, the Czech Republic and Poland, Popic's work illuminates the factors and mechanisms accounting for such cross-country variation. Challenging existing interpretations in the literature, the volume conceptualizes policy change as an endogenous process based on "learning", thus leading the reader to a fascinating journey into how the never-ending "ballet" between Ideas, institutions and parties shaped the politics of reform and, ultimately, policy outputs."

—Matteo Jessoula, *University of Milan, Italy*

"Tamara Popic's Health reforms in Post-Communist Eastern Europe offers us deep insights into how neo-liberal ideas were translated into real health reforms in Eastern Europe after the fall of communism. Popic shows how ideas were translated into specific policy trajectories in different institutional and historical contexts. This excellent book demonstrates not only that ideas are important, but also how and why policy ideas evolve. Popic's theory of policy learning offers deep insights into both the evolution of health policies in several countries and why we see such different policy outcomes in different societies. This well written book will be of interest to anyone interested in the ways in which ideas, institutions and policy legacies interact over time"

—Sven Steinmo, *University of Colorado, Boulder, CO, USA*

Tamara Popic

Health Reforms in Post-Communist Eastern Europe

The Politics of Policy Learning

palgrave
macmillan

Tamara Popic
School of Politics and International Relations
Queen Mary University of London
London, UK

ISBN 978-3-031-15499-7 ISBN 978-3-031-15497-3 (eBook)
https://doi.org/10.1007/978-3-031-15497-3

This Palgrave Macmillan imprint is published by the registered company Springer Nature Switzerland AG.
The registered company address is: Gewerbestrasse 11, 6330 Cham, Switzerland

To Lorenzo and David

About the Book

This book provides the first in-depth study of healthcare reform in post-communist Eastern Europe. Combining insights from comparative politics and public policy analysis, it examines health reforms in Slovenia, the Czech Republic, and Poland between 1989 and 2019. The book argues that the transformation of post-communist health systems has entailed a process of policy learning and that the pathways taken by different states away from communist-era healthcare system have been shaped by a series of reform initiatives aimed at adapting of market-oriented policy ideas in healthcare provision. The success of these initiatives has been influenced by three factors: policy legacies, political competition, and institutional configurations. The book offers a novel and important comparison of health reform in the region, as well as policy changes more generally. It will appeal to scholars and students of public policy, health policy, and European politics.

Acknowledgements

This book would not have been possible without people who provided inspiration, encouragement or other types of support for its research and writing. Its 'beginnings' date back to 2009, when I enrolled in the doctoral programme at the European University Institute (EUI) and was given an opportunity to pick a topic of my choice for my PhD research. My gratitude goes first and foremost to Sven Steinmo for his generous support and guidance as I was developing my first ideas about the politics of health reforms in post-communism. I am also very grateful to Ellen Immergut, for the stimulating intellectual support and comments which provided inspiring motivation as I worked on the book during my postdoc period. Ellen was also incredibly generous with her advice on different aspects of the book publishing and writing, and I feel deeply indebted to her for helping me with the first steps in finding a balance between academia and motherhood, two worlds that I combined as I started writing the book. I am also grateful to my colleagues from the Max Weber Programme's Writers Group—Bilyana Petrova, Takuya Onoda, and Alexandru Moise—who provided highly stimulating comments on the book's first draft chapters and encouraged its further writing. I also thank Diana Burlacu, my colleague and co-author, for sharp comments on book's contribution. At my new academic 'home', Queen Mary University of London, I am very grateful to David Williams for the understanding and time he generously provided—both were needed to finalize this book.

Furthermore, I am grateful to Nick Barclay, who accepted my book proposal for Palgrave Macmillan, and to Karthika Devi and the rest of the Palgrave production team for their support and patience. I am also very grateful to the anonymous reviewer who was encouragingly enthusiastic about the book's proposal, provided a set of insightful comments and approved the final version of the manuscript. I further thank Elizabeth Thompson for her careful copy-editing, and Marija Jankovic together with Primer Studio for generously helping me produce the image for the cover of the book.

On a personal level, I am deeply indebted to my close friends and colleagues, Jelena Dzankic, Nevena Kulic, Visnja Vukov and Simone Tholens, who provided crucial support and encouragement in the final phases of the book writing. Finally, I am deeply grateful for the support of my parents, Jovan and Ljubinka, and my sister Jovana. I owe the most to my father Jovan who was the first to trigger my intellectual curiosity and has always been a great source of moral support for my academic efforts. The very final and the deepest gratitude goes to my life partner Lorenzo and son David, for their patience as they lived the writing of this book as a daily effort, but were also the greatest source of joy throughout the process. I dedicate this book to the two of them.

Contents

About the Author

Tamara Popic is Lecturer in Social/Public Policy at the School of Politics and International Relations, Queen Mary University of London, UK. Her research interests include health politics and policy in post-communist countries. She is the co-editor of *Health Policy in Europe: A Handbook* (2021).

Abbreviations

ANO 211:	Action of Dissatisfied Citizens (Czech Republic)
AWS:	Solidarity Election Action (Poland)
CPI:	Complementary private insurance (Slovenia)
ČSSD:	Czech Social Democratic Party (Czech Republic)
DeSUS:	Democratic Party of Pensioners of Slovenia (Slovenia)
DL:	Civic List (Slovenia)
GHIF:	General Health Insurance Fund (Czech Republic)
HIF:	Health Insurance Fund (Czech Republic)
HIIS:	Health Insurance Institute of Slovenia (Slovenia)
KDS:	Christian Democratic Party (Czech Republic)
KDU-ČSL:	Coalition of Christian and Democratic Union and Czechoslovak People's Party (Czech Republic)
KLD:	Liberal Democratic Congress (Poland)
KLS:	Christian's People Party (Slovenia)
KSČM:	Communist Party of Bohemia and Moravia (Czech Republic)
LDS:	Liberal Democratic Party (Slovenia)
LOK-SČL:	Doctor's Trade Union Club (Czech Republic)
LPR:	League of Polish Families (Poland)
NFZ:	National Health Fund (Poland)
NHS:	National Health Service
NSi:	New Slovenia—Christian Democrats (Slovenia)
ODS:	Civic Democratic Party (Czech Republic)
OFZ:	Civic Forum of Health Professionals (Czech Republic)
OSA:	Civic Democratic Alliance (Czech Republic)
PChD:	Party of Christian Democrats (Poland)
PiS:	Law and Justice (Poland)
PO:	Civic Platform (Poland)

PPPP:	Polish Beer Lovers' Party (Poland)
PS:	Positive Slovenia (Slovenia)
PSL-PL:	Polish People's Party (Poland)
PZPR:	Polish United Workers Party (Poland)
SD:	Social Democrats (Slovenia)
SdRP:	Social Democracy of the Republic of Poland (Poland)
SDS:	Slovenian Democratic Party (Slovenia)
SDSS/SDS:	Social Democratic Party (Slovenia)
SFRY:	Socialist Federal Republic of Yugoslavia
SHI:	Social Health Insurance
SKD:	Christian Democrats (Slovenia)
SLD:	Democratic Left Alliance (Poland)
SLS:	Slovene People's Party (Slovenia)
SMC:	Modern Centre Party (Slovenia)
SPP:	Slovenian People's Party (Slovenia)
SPZOZ:	Autonomous Public Healthcare Units (Poland)
SRP:	Self-Defence of the Republic of Poland (Poland)
SZ:	Green Party (Czech Republic)
TOP09:	Tradition, Responsibility, Prosperity (Czech Republic)
UD:	Democratic Union (Poland)
UP:	Labour Union (Poland)
US-DEU:	Freedom Union-Democratic Union (Czech Republic)
UW:	Freedom Union (Poland)
VV:	Public Affairs (Czech Republic)
WB:	World Bank
WHO:	World Health Organisation
ZARES:	Social Liberals (Slovenia)
ZKS:	League of Communists (Slovenia)
SD:	Social Democrats (Slovenia)
ZcHN:	Christian National Union (Poland)
ZLSD:	United List of Social Democrats (Slovenia)
ZOZ:	Healthcare Unit (Poland)
ZSMS:	Federation of the Socialist Youth of Slovenia (Slovenia)

List of Tables

CHAPTER 1

Introduction

Introduction

Writing about a highly controversial health law in the Czech Republic, a 2008 article in *The New York Times* reported the introduction of patient fees for medical services, including a fee of $1.85 to see a doctor. Clearly puzzled by how such a small fee could generate so much public outrage, the journalist suggested healthcare was a sensitive issue in the Czech Republic and, indeed, in Eastern Europe more generally. 'The idea of charging anything for healthcare can generate significant controversy', he pointed out, 'because many Czechs see it as a matter of principle that healthcare should be free' (*New York Times* 2008).

As this book goes on to show, the introduction of user fees during post-communist health reforms in the Eastern Bloc countries was one of many measures that marked a departure from the state-dominated system of healthcare in which medical services were provided centrally and hierarchically, but also universally, at no cost to citizens. Emerging out of the communist era, however, these systems had numerous problems and in the context of the double transition to capitalism and democracy, policymakers looked to private markets and competition, hoping this would improve the efficiency and quality of healthcare provision, as well as eradicate ubiquitous corruption.

Of course, post-communist countries were not alone in this: attempts to reduce public funding for healthcare, shifting to a mix of public and

T. Popic, *Health Reforms in Post-Communist Eastern Europe*,
https://doi.org/10.1007/978-3-031-15497-3_1

private funding and replacing state with market mechanisms in the provision of medical services, entered European governments' health reform agendas in the 1990s (Immergut et al. 2021a; see also Tritter et al. 2009; Thomson et al. 2009; Gingrich 2011). Yet in the Eastern Bloc, these market-oriented tendencies were particularly strong, as after almost 50 years of the state-dominated, socialist command-and-control systems of healthcare based on central planning, newly democratic governments embraced markets and privatisation with enthusiasm. Eastern European countries, as shown in this book, essentially became laboratories testing market-oriented ideas and their adaptation to the post-communist health context.

Healthcare reforms in the three countries discussed in this book (Poland, Slovenia, and Czech Republic) are interesting comparative cases of the turn to markets. In the Czech Republic, beside the above-mentioned user fees, the government introduced a highly market-oriented, competitive insurance system and installed a reimbursement method for doctors' services based on a competitive fee-for-service model that, far from working as planned, actually generated textbook examples of market failure. In Slovenia, one of the main aspects of the breakdown of the socialist model was the introduction of co-payments for healthcare and complementary private health insurance, and these became an integral part of the new health system. In Poland, market enthusiasm led to radical but failed market reforms in the early transition, followed by continuous efforts to push for further marketisation through various measures, including the transformation of public hospitals into private, for-profit commercial companies. Whilst these market reforms were embraced enthusiastically by the post-communist policymakers, they also generated criticism and inspired heated debates revolving around substantial social values of egalitarianism, fairness, and solidarity.

The examples of market-oriented health reforms in the Eastern Bloc are illustrative of a much wider departure from, in principle, a very generous 'cradle-to-grave' system of social benefits built under socialism. This welfare system developed gradually during the post-war period and was labelled a 'premature welfare state', characterised by universal entitlements out of proportion with countries' resources and fiscal capacity (Kornai 1997). Ending socialism whilst still adhering to some of the core values of the welfare state, such as universalism, was a notable challenge for the new democratic leaders in the Eastern Bloc. Economic transition led to restructuring, generating radical disruptions, crises, and unexpectedly high social costs (Standing 1996; Milanovic 2014; Ghodsee and Orenstein 2021). Moreover, the remaking of the welfare state in these burgeoning democracies took place in the context of party system development, institution building, and, in some cases, state-building and, as such, was a laborious process of 're-building the ship at sea' (Elster et al. 1998).

Against this background, the book focuses on a relatively understudied area of the post-communist welfare restructuring: healthcare reforms. Most attention in work on the post-communist welfare state has been dedicated to another large social policy sector—pensions—with researchers showing how policy models have differed across countries (see Orenstein 2008; Armeanu 2010; Guardiancich 2012; Sokhey 2017). This book points to a similar pattern of cross-country differences in healthcare policy, noting the puzzling variations in the success of specific, market-oriented health reforms. As a closer look at health reforms across the Eastern Bloc countries reveals, although attempts to push for reforms to privatise and marketise healthcare were similar, countries took different paths to reform. Whilst in some cases, governments remodelled the healthcare system from a public, state-dominated model to a private, market-oriented system relatively easily, in others, they tried hard but had mixed results, and in still others, the healthcare system shows very few signs of change, suggesting all government efforts have been for naught.

The book provides the first in-depth analysis of the variety in the healthcare reforms across Eastern Europe by looking at three exemplary cases: Slovenia, Poland, and Czech Republic.[1] Building on the concept of ideationally driven, endogenous policy change, its key claim is that the transformation of the post-communist health systems essentially entailed a process of learning. Eastern European policymakers sought to marketise and privatise their healthcare systems through a series of reform initiatives aimed at solving policy problems, in what in retrospect can be seen as a trial and error process. This process of policy learning was driven by ideas rooted in the belief that market mechanisms such as competition and privatisation would solve the problems of the healthcare system, yielding higher efficiency and better allocation of resources. The policy learning entailed not only gaining an understanding of how to adjust

[1] Studies of the post-communist welfare restructuring that cover healthcare are either restricted to very brief descriptions of some of the aspects of healthcare system transformations (see Kuitto 2016) or offer short cross-country comparisons (see Szikra and Tomka 2009).

market-oriented ideas to healthcare and tailor them to specific policy problems, but also figuring out how to transform these ideas into actual policies. This process of learning, or 'puzzling through' (see Heclo 1974), was decisively shaped by individual countries' health policy legacies, institutions, and dynamics of political party competition.

The rest of the chapter proceeds as follows. It first defines the core concept of the book, healthcare markets, and then offers a brief overview of health reforms across the post-communist region, highlighting the considerable variation. This discussion sets the stage for the book's main research question: What explains the variation in health policy trajectories of market-oriented health reforms across the post-communist countries in Eastern Europe? The chapter touches on the Czech, Slovenian, and Polish post-communist health policy paths and briefly shows how countries' individual differences in health policy legacies, institutions, and political party competition explain the differences between the three cases. The chapter then lists the book's contributions to the literature, explains the method and data collection, and concludes with an outline of the book, summarising the content of each chapter.

Market-Oriented Health Reforms

As mentioned earlier, the introduction of markets in healthcare was not a uniquely post-socialist phenomenon. In the last several decades, countries across Europe have introduced some sort of market mechanism into the financing and delivery of medical services. Yet, markets in healthcare represent a complex policy phenomenon, partly because healthcare, like welfare sectors more generally, is considered particularly prone to market failure (Arrow 1963; Barr 2004). This section discusses some of the core issues surrounding markets in healthcare and gives an overview of two dimensions of these markets: conceptual and historical.

Some of the core theoretical discussions around markets in healthcare come from the field of microeconomics. From this point of view, issues with healthcare markets emerge because healthcare is a welfare sector especially likely to experience market failure. The free market is considered not suitable for healthcare because the need for healthcare goods and services is unpredictable, and individuals have considerable difficulty making decisions that are in their own interests because of the specific character of these goods and services, and this in turn, leads to market failures (Arrow 1963). Most of these failures are information related and centre on knowledge asymmetries in the relationship between doctor and patient, between doctor and payer, and between purchasers of insurance and insurance companies. These failures lead to the general view that assigning a central role to private and competitive market forces is not a particularly efficient way to run a health system; hence, markets are not as good as state, i.e. public system in providing healthcare. This view is held even by some of the most liberal economists (see Hayek 2007).[2]

The economic issues aside, what are healthcare markets? How can we best define them? The definitions in the literature are mixed. For example, these markets can be defined with reference to the broader phenomenon of markets in the welfare state. 'The chief feature that distinguishes markets from other forms of organization', according to Gingrich, 'is that they influence behaviour manipulating incentives for consumers and producers of services' (Gingrich 2011: 7–8). This definition is useful in that it distinguishes markets from both the hierarchical 'command-and-control' systems, in which a central agency defines processes and outcomes, and from 'network' systems, in which users and providers operate on the basis of trust (Gingrich 2011).

There are other, more specific definitions of markets in the healthcare sector. Julian Le Grand, one of the founding fathers of the market-oriented reforms in the British health system under the Tony Blair government, defined market-oriented mechanisms of healthcare provision not as 'pure' markets but as 'quasi-markets' (Le Grand and Bartlett 1993; Le Grand 2011). In 'quasi-markets', services are provided by competitive providers, just as in pure markets, but the purchasers of those services are financed by state resources, not private ones. Similar to 'quasi-markets' in education, for example, 'quasi markets' in healthcare imply services are free or largely free at the point of delivery; unlike most forms of state provision, the user has a choice of provider, and the providers themselves operate in a competitive market (Le Grand 2011: 80–81).

Tracking market-oriented changes in healthcare, other authors have distinguished between the 'economisation' and 'marketisation' of healthcare. Ewert (2009), for example, argued there is a significant difference

[2] According to Hayek: 'Whereas in the case of sickness and accident, neither the desire to avoid such calamities nor the efforts to overcome their consequences are as a rule weakened by the provision of assistance—where, in short, we deal with genuinely insurable risks—the case for the state's helping to organize a comprehensive system of social insurance is very strong' (Hayek 2007: 148).

between the two processes in the degree to which they attach importance to the state. Whilst ‘economised’ health policy depends on a strong and regulative state and involves elements of central steering, ‘marketisation’ reduces the impact of the state by initiating competition between non-profit and for-profit providers, contracting-out certain services, or forming new kinds of contracts between users and providers, without the state (Ewert 2009: 24).

This book combines these different conceptualisations to define the healthcare markets introduced in the post-communist context. Building on the definition of health markets as ‘quasi-markets’ (Le Grand 2011), instruments that combine elements of state funding of healthcare with consumer choice and competition, it pays attention to the behavioural dimension of markets in healthcare. As shown throughout the book, the introduction of market mechanisms in the post-communist countries essentially implied a shift from the ‘command-and-control’ model in which the state as a central agency had exclusive control of the provision of the medical services (see Gingrich 2011). In this model, healthcare facilities belonged to the state, medical professionals were state employees on fixed salaries and patients’ access to care was territorially determined and hence restricted (Field 1991). Healthcare was financed according to a main instrument of classical socialism, a ‘Five Year Plan’, with a pre-established share of the state budget dedicated to the sector (Weinerman 1969). In this context, the post-communist shift to a ‘market-oriented’ healthcare system, the term used here, implied the introduction of new mechanisms of healthcare provision, or ‘marketisation’, which aimed at changing incentives for consumers and producers of health services (Gingrich 2011), with countries taking different routes to the reduction of the state’s role in healthcare (see Ewert 2009).

In terms of healthcare financing, the introduction of healthcare markets meant a reduction of public funding and an increase in private ‘out-of-pocket’ payments for health services. In terms of healthcare delivery, it involved the conversion of public, state-owned healthcare facilities into private, either non- or for-profit organisations, in some instances, subject to commercial rather than public law. More essentially, however, this reduction in the role of the state aimed to influence the behaviour of the main actors in the sector by changing incentives for patients as consumers and for providers as producers of health services. Patients became able to choose their own doctors or insurance funds and change them if they were not satisfied. Through other market measures, such as user fees or co-payments for services, patients were incentivised to change their approach to the use of health services. For their part, doctors found they had new incentives driving their service provision, and this depended on the methods used to reimburse them for their services, implying less (e.g. capitation) or more (e.g. fee-for-service) competition amongst providers. Taken together, these new incentives meant that in the post-communist context, healthcare provision provided a new playing field for both patients as users and doctors as producers of services, establishing a very different context of healthcare provision than the state-led one.

From a historical perspective, markets in healthcare are certainly not an invention of the twentieth century. Use of markets to deliver healthcare can be traced to the early developments of the European healthcare systems in the eighteenth century (Immergut et al. 2021a). However, in the 1970s and 1980s, in the context of advanced industrial democracies and universal welfare states, the interest in markets took on a new energy (Callahan and Wasunna 2006; Tritter et al. 2009). The emergence of markets in healthcare coincided with a period of the 1970s economic crisis, when calls for prudent government spending were heard in a number of European countries. By the 1980s, many policymakers across Europe were advocates of healthcare markets, but it was in the United Kingdom, under Margaret Thatcher's Conservative government, where markets won their first major political battle (Giaimo 2009). Thatcher's government opted for a series of reforms introducing 'internal markets' into the healthcare system (Gingrich 2011; Gingrich and Greer 2021). Affection for markets spread quickly amongst policymakers in the rest of Western Europe. Governments gradually introduced markets in healthcare, hoping this would significantly improve the financial sustainability of a sector increasingly challenged by the growing costs of care and the changing healthcare needs of the population.

In the 1990s, there was a dramatic upsurge in the scale and character of market-oriented initiatives in healthcare systems across Europe (see Immergut et al. 2021a). A variety of market-inspired attempts to stimulate innovations in service provision appeared in- and outside the public healthcare sector, including increased quality and greater efficiency, as market mechanisms started to be used in the provision of both core and ancillary healthcare services. A common orientation towards the market became evident in all European countries, despite the peculiarity of the historical and structural differences between their healthcare systems, such as those between the National Health Service (NHS) and the Social Health Insurance (SHI) systems.[3]

The Nordic countries—Sweden, Norway, and Denmark—all known for their NHS tradition, with strongly universal state-led health systems built during the post-war period, gradually introduced various market elements in publicly financed healthcare, including increased patient choice and privatisation of primary care (Blomqvist and Winblad 2021; Schoyen 2021; Larsen and Stone 2015). Similarly, in the Netherlands and Germany, where healthcare provision is based on SHI systems, managed competition, profit-making providers, and increased out-of-pocket payments became commonly used tools of healthcare provision (see Anderson and Van Druenen 2021; Immergut and Wendt 2021). Finally, in South European countries, such as Italy, Spain, and Portugal, where NHS-style universal health systems were established more recently, markets found a place in healthcare in elements such as private health insurance and public–private partnerships (Maino and Razetti 2021; Chuliá 2021; Asensio 2021). Because of this pan-European move towards markets, the decades following the 1990s saw a substantial re-configuration of the healthcare sector, strongly characterised by an increase in market-oriented activities in financing, organisation, delivery, and management of healthcare provision (see Saltman and Figueras 1997; Saltman et al. 2004).

It is also worth noting that the introduction of markets in healthcare across Europe was accompanied by changes in policy discourse. A new emphasis on terms such as 'individual responsibility', 'choice', and 'consumers', replaced the old policy rhetoric focusing on universal, public, and solidarity-based healthcare provision, even in countries with a long tradition of healthcare provided in a state-led system (see Tritter et al. 2009). In Sweden, the political parties in power in the 1990s called for a 'freedom of choice revolution' that would empower the dependent clients of state services by transforming them into self-confident customers (Rothstein 1998). Almost simultaneously, the Conservative government's policy discourse in the United Kingdom challenged the entrenched, inefficient and unresponsive public services in healthcare and re-conceptualised patients as consumers, encouraging them to be demanding (Light 2003). As this book goes on to show, the introduction of market-oriented health policies

[3]The traditional distinction between the NHS (also called 'Beveridge') and SHI ('Bismarck') systems is that whilst the former are funded by taxes, that is, state budgets, the latter are funded by workers' compulsory contributions to health insurance (see Toth 2021).

in the Eastern Bloc was accompanied by a similar change at the level of policy discourse, with terms such 'individual responsibility' or 'healthcare consumer' becoming part of governments' framing of policy change.

Whilst the discourse surrounding market reforms was similar in Eastern and Western Europe, one significant difference in market-oriented and more general health reforms in the two regions should be noted. In the East, healthcare reforms, at least initially, had a different set of objectives (see Bartlett et al. 2012). The post-communist healthcare sectors were plagued by underfunding, shortages, and corruption, with hordes of poorly paid doctors and unsatisfied patients (Cockerham 2002; Kornai and Eggleston 2001). In this context, in stark contrast to Western Europe where market-oriented reforms were used to improve the financial sustainability of the sector and basically cut public funding, in the Eastern Bloc, they were seen as a way of bringing more money into the public system and more generally, as a way to improve funding for the healthcare sector as a whole. This explains why, for example, despite external advice not to introduce the SHI model in the early economic transition because it did not incorporate state control of spending, the Czech and Slovenian post-communist reformers determinedly went against this advice (see Chaps. 3 and 4). Gradually, however, the objectives of the post-communist health reforms came closer to those in the West, with calls for sector sustainability through austerity peaking in the context of the global financial crisis.

Healthcare Reforms in Post-Communism

Analytically, the post-communist reforms can be divided into two parallel streams. The first was a whole-region, systemic shift from the National Health Service (NHS) style health system in which healthcare is funded by taxes, that is, the state budget, in the region labeled as the Soviet 'Semashko system',[4] to a Social Health Insurance (SHI) or 'Bismarck' system in which healthcare is funded by insurance contributions (see Marrée and Groenewegen 1997). The second was the introduction of a wide range of market-oriented policy instruments in both financing and healthcare delivery, with varying paths and outcomes.

[4]Semashko system was named after Nikolai Semashko, People's Commissar of Public Health in the Soviet Russia (1918–1930).

Systemic Change: From 'Semashko' to 'Bismarck'

During the first post-communist decade, the Soviet-style NHS 'Semashko' system of healthcare was replaced with the 'Bismarck' system based on social health insurance (SHI) (Marrée and Groenewegen 1997).[5] The shift to the SHI model left one of the characteristics of communist healthcare provision in place, namely universal access to healthcare, but changed its overall organisational logic. The most important changes were the separation of the two previously integrated system functions, financing and delivery of healthcare services, and the introduction of new institutions responsible for healthcare funding: healthcare insurance funds.

In healthcare financing, insurance contributions in the form of payroll taxes replaced general taxation as the main source of healthcare funding. These contributions became mandatory, based on employment, and were defined as percentages of workers' salaries. Another novelty in financing was the introduction of health insurance funds; these were established as bodies responsible for the collection and administration of the insurance contributions and the purchasing of medical services from healthcare providers.

In healthcare delivery, organisational and institutional changes were equally wide-ranging. After the dissolution of the centralised and hierarchical system of healthcare facilities, the delivery system was transformed in such a way that healthcare facilities gained the status of individual entities responsible for the delivery of different types of care. As individual entities, facilities became independent from the state and were granted a considerable degree of administrative and financial autonomy. Similarly, doctors who were previously the employees of the state became able to practice medicine independently.

Policy Change: Introduction of Markets

Healthcare policy under communism provided care according to the 'command-and-control' model of healthcare provision, whereby the delivery and financing of healthcare services were state-dominated, centralised, and hierarchical. Health policy was an integral part of the socialist command economy and, as such, was in line with the economic mechanism of 'classical socialism', similar to the other policy sectors of the socialist state (Kornai 1992). Resources dedicated to healthcare were relatively modest, as

[5] Slovenia was an exception; it was the only Central Eastern European country to keep the social health insurance system) during the post-war period (see Chap. 3), which implied that it did not shift from NHS to SHI system in the post-communist period.

healthcare was not considered an important part of the socialist economy and was therefore given low priority. These resources were distributed according to a very centralised and hierarchical scheme fully controlled by the state, so that the governance of healthcare resources was based on a very strict top-down decision-making logic (see Kornai and Eggleston 2001).[6]

The departure from this state-dominated healthcare policy model was initiated in the immediate aftermath of the fall of communism. The 'shift to the SHI, Bismarckian' system allowed for specific separation of healthcare financing from delivery, which played an important role in this departure, as it enabled policymakers to introduce a wide range of market instruments in both dimensions of healthcare provision.[7] In healthcare financing, these instruments were create through policies introducing co-payments, user fees (flat fees) for healthcare goods and services, and voluntary private health insurance, thus breaking away from the fully-funded public model of healthcare and partially transferring healthcare costs to patients. Marketisation of financing also involved the rejection of the hierarchical model of resource distribution, and the introduction of competitive healthcare insurance purchasing mechanism such as selective contracting, and various forms of competitive compensation schemes for healthcare providers, establishing the so-called 'managed competition' in the insurance sector. Similarly, marketisation in healthcare delivery involved privatisation of healthcare facilities, with the transfer of healthcare facilities from state to private hands, mainly in primary, but also increasingly in hospital care. These measures were also accompanied with the departure from territorially determined access to healthcare, and the introduction of patient choice (Table 1.1).

Following Gingrich's (Gingrich 2011) definition of markets, it is possible to talk about a 'family resemblance' between these different forms of markets introduced into the post-communist healthcare, as all forms used competitive mechanisms to allocate scarce resources, manipulating the behavioural incentives of the main actors in the health system. Yet, if we look more carefully at the post-communist reform trajectories, it is also possible to distinguish country-specific paths towards healthcare markets. While some countries showed continuity, introducing and keeping

[6] Slovenia moved away from this centralized model of healthcare earlier than the other countries in the Eastern Bloc, through a shift to worker 'self-management' in the 1970s (see Chap. 3).

[7] The SHI system was introduced in all the countries, except Latvia, in the following year: Croatia (1993); Czech Republic (1991); Bulgaria (1998); Estonia (1991), Hungary (1988): Lithuania (1996); Poland (1997); Serbia (1992); Slovakia (1992); Slovenia (1992).

Table 1.1 Market-oriented healthcare reforms in post-communist countries (1989–2019)[a]

Country/ Dimension	*Healthcare financing*	*Healthcare delivery*
Croatia	Voluntary private health insurance (1993), withdrawal (2001) Co-payments (2001) User fees (2005)	Privatisation of primary care (1993)
Czech Republic	Managed competition (1991, 1992), regulation (1995, 1996) User fees (2007), withdrawal (2014)	Privatisation of primary care (1992) Hospital privatisation (1997), withdrawal (2006) and re-introduction (2011)
Bulgaria	User fees (1998) Managed competition, failed attempt (2008) Selective contracting (2015)	Privatisation of primary care (1991); Hospital privatisation (1999), withdrawal (2002) and re-introduction (2008), failed attempt (2015)
Estonia	Co-payments (1995) Selective contracting (2002)	Privatisation of primary care (2001)
Hungary	Co-payments (2006)	Privatisation of primary care (1989) Hospital privatisation (2001)
Latvia	Co-payments (1995)	Hospital privatisation (2000)
Lithuania	Co-payments (1996)	Privatisation of primary care (1995)
Poland	Managed competition (1998), withdrawal (2003)	Privatisation of primary care (1991) Hospital privatisation (2008), withdrawal (2008), re-introduction (2011)
Serbia	Co-payments (2005)	Privatisation of primary care (1989) Hospital privatisation (2005)
Slovakia	Co-payments (2003) Managed competition (2004), withdrawal (2006), re-introduction (2011) User fees (2004), withdrawal (2006, 2015)	Privatisation of primary care (1994) Hospital privatisation (2001, 2006), withdrawal (2007)
Slovenia	Co-payments (1992) Voluntary private health insurance (1993)	Privatisation of primary care (1992)

Source: Author's elaboration based on Immergut et al. (2021a, b)

[a]While this table covers mainly market-oriented reforms, for broader overview of reforms for the same period, see Immergut et al. (2021)

markets elements in provision of medical services, others featured more turbulent reforms, experiencing policy withdrawals and renewed attempts to re-install policies aimed on shifting away from the state-led system.

Explaining the Variation in Post-Communist Health Reforms: Argument

A closer look at the cross-country analysis reveals considerable variations in the healthcare policy paths of post-communist countries over three transitional decades. These variations are best illustrated by the trajectories of market reforms in three countries covered in this book—Slovenia, the Czech Republic, and Poland. As the book goes on to show, in each of the three countries, policymakers intensively sought to introduce market instruments in healthcare, but they did so with varying degrees of success and, even when they were successful, their reforms did not always stand the test of time. In Slovenia, this path was marked by *survival*, as the policy introduced in the early transition stood the test of time over the three communist decades. The Czech health policy path displayed *instability*, as market elements were introduced but then partially withdrawn. Lastly, in Poland, healthcare policy showed radical *reversals* that in comparison to the policy of the other two countries, more closely resembled state-dominated healthcare provision.

The variation might not be surprising. A close look at the three decades of reforms reveals a nuanced picture of unique, country-specific health policy successes and failures. Yet, the main argument of this book is not that the post-communist health reforms varied across countries and over time. Rather, the core claim is that this variation was the result of different learning processes. Eastern European policymakers sought to marketise and privatise their healthcare systems through a series of reform initiatives aimed at solving policy problems by relying on market-oriented ideas. However, the post-communist health reforms did not involve a simple translation of these market ideas into policy. Nor did they imply that the countries' policy paths varied because of the influence of professional interests, external actors, or economic pressures. Rather, the reform trajectories varied because of the differences in individual countries' previous experiences with markets in healthcare under socialism, institutional configurations under democracy, and political party competition.

Pre-transitional policy legacies—in particular, experience with non-state mechanisms of health provision under communism—proved crucial for the successful transformation of ideas into policy in the early transition. Policymakers' experiences with such mechanisms reduced the risk of reform failures and facilitated the learning process in its crucial initial phase. The transformation of market ideas into policy was also shaped by institutional configurations. Made up of formal constitutional rules, these configurations defined veto points at which reform proposals could be blocked in the policymaking process; this created constraints but also opportunities for policy learning by influencing the strategies of the reformers. Lastly, the transformation of ideas into policy was also shaped by the dynamics of political competition. This affected party positions on health policy, and these, in turn, shaped patterns of political support for and opposition to market ideas, channelled through institutional configurations.

More specifically, in Slovenia, previous policy experiences with competition and privatisation in healthcare under socialism allowed policymakers to implement carefully-thought-out, cautious reforms at the beginning of the transition. Thanks to this positive initial experience, Slovenian policymakers quickly gained an understanding of how to adjust market mechanisms to healthcare and tailor them to policy problems at hand. Further market reforms were facilitated by a relatively loose network of veto points and a lack of major partisan division over health policy, all of which generated opportunities for adjustments.

As they lacked previous experience with markets, the initial learning process of the Czech policymakers was more troublesome. Early transitional reforms provided some textbook examples of market failures, but led to a recognition of the need for market regulation. Relatively soft but nevertheless persistent partisan division over health policy, in combination with a light veto point structure, subsequently generated a protracted learning process that involved the use of political strategies aimed at overcoming institutional constraints to intended health reforms.

In Poland, as in the Czech Republic, the first attempts at healthcare reform based on market ideas went astray due to a lack of previous experience. Moreover, sharp partisan division over the course of reforms led to policy reversals, preventing Polish policymakers from learning from their negative initial experience. A combination of divisive political dynamics and institutional configurations beset with many veto points subsequently continued to generate reform-and-reversal patterns in Polish healthcare policy, disrupting the learning process.

The main argument of this book challenges the dominant view of post-communist healthcare restructuring as essentially shaped by professional interests, external factors, or economic pressures (see Chap. 2). The book claims that reforming post-communist healthcare involved an endogenous process of policy change which originated in the socialist period, when market-oriented ideas emerged in response to the anomalies of the socialist healthcare model. By explaining the variation in post-communist healthcare policy paths as policy learning—adaptations of similar policy ideas in different political contexts—the argument accounts for why, in some contexts, these ideas translated into policy and in others they did not, despite the efforts of policymakers. In short, the book points out that we need to look at politics, or more specifically, how factors such as legacies, institutional structures, and political party competition shape policymakers' attempts to translate ideas into policy.

The book's argument also offers new perspectives with respect to traditional views of the influence of legacies, institutions and parties on policymaking. For legacies, it shows that it is not the legacies *per se*, but rather the perception of previous policy experiences that shapes the reform process (see Bohle and Greskovits 2012). For institutions, the book shows that although institutional veto configurations impose important constraints on the policymaking process (Immergut 1992), it is the combination of these configurations with the dynamics generated by party competition that helps explain why governments are able to pass certain reforms but not others (see Popic 2021). For party politics, the book's findings suggest the traditional party divisions into left and right are often of little use in understanding the politics of health (see Tavits and Letki 2009). Instead, the more specific divisions over health issues should be analysed within the broader context of party competition, which in the post-communist context featured dynamic processes of party transformation and identity building (see Chap. 2).

Data and Methods

Data used in this book come from official policy documents, transcripts of parliamentary debates, legislative bills discussed and/or approved in the national parliaments, and newspaper articles collected for the three decades (1989–2019) on health reforms in the analysed countries. The original research materials also included thirty in-depth interviews conducted with key players in the reform processes. These were conducted as semi-structured interviews focused on the reforms of the post-communist period, and interviewees included key informants, experts, and decision makers (for a list of the interviewees, see the Appendix).

Methodologically, the book relies on a small-N qualitative approach. The small-N approach is a case-oriented research strategy focused upon a small number of cases, analysed with attention to each case as an interpretable whole (Ragin 2000). Importantly for the purposes of this book, this method reflects the specificity of each case, but allows for historically concrete generalisations (Della Porta and Keating 2008). The particular research technique used for the assessment of each case was process tracing. This technique involves the identification of steps in a causal process leading to the outcome of a given dependent variable of a particular case (Beach and Pedersen 2013; Bennett and Checkel 2015). The technique is particularly suitable for intensive case studies; it allows an inductive approach to be combined with a causal-analytical framework. More precisely, it makes it possible to analyse which dimensions of policy legacies, institutions, and party competition figured in policy change and how. This approach allows for identification of elements of policy change, that is, a specific policy outcome (or lack thereof), and for going 'backward from the outcome by sifting through the evidence in an attempt to uncover a plausible sufficient causal mechanism that produced the outcome' (Beach and Pedersen 2013: 169).

Overview of the Book

The rest of this book is structured as follows. Chapter 2 develops the central argument of the book—the claim that the variation in heath policy trajectories across Eastern Bloc countries during the first three decades of transition reflects differences in the processes of policy learning, driven by ideas and shaped by historical, political, and institutional factors. The first part of the chapter locates this argument within the comparative public policy literature which understands policymaking as a learning process driven by ideas and also provides an analytical framework of policy learning linking ideas with the outputs of the policymaking (Fig. 2.1). The second part of the chapter develops the argument by concentrating on factors shaping the policy learning process. It first accounts for the role of legacies by showing how past policy experiences with state and market mechanisms of health provision inherited from the communist period influenced the first post-communist attempts at policy reform. Next, it looks at the role of institutional veto configurations (Table 2.1) and explains how a combination of these configurations and the dynamics of political competition influenced the learning process in the new Eastern European democracies, formalising this part of the argument in a table (Table 3.1). The chapter also contrasts this core argument of the book with the existing explanations which see healthcare reforms as the result of professional power, the influence of external actors, or global economic pressures. The chapter concludes by summarising the argument, setting the scene for the in-depth empirical analyses of the three case studies.

Chapter 3 provides evidence for the Slovenian case. It demonstrates how a combination of favourable legacies, institutional configurations, and non-divisive politics allowed a relatively smooth learning process in which market ideas, although challenged, displayed remarkable resilience in the development of health policy. The chapter starts by providing background on the country's healthcare system under communism and the political context of the early transition. It stresses the role of Slovenia's previous policy experiences with social health insurance and self-management—a guiding principle of healthcare system organisation under communism—as key factors in policy learning in this early phase. A progressive learning process was further fuelled by a lack of partisan division over health policy between the two main political parties, the successfully transformed communist successor party, Social Democrats (ZLSD/SD), and the Liberals (LDS), and by a relatively light structure of institutional constraints. The core of the chapter comprises a chronology of the four most relevant market-oriented health reforms during the post-communist period. It shows how the early transition health reforms under the LDS-led government (1992, 1993) privatised the country's healthcare financing by introducing co-payments for medical services and complementary private insurance (CPI). This introduction of CPI stood in stark contrast to the policymakers' decision to significantly limit the privatisation of primary care and to keep Slovenian hospitals in public hands, suggesting a rather cautious approach to markets in health thanks largely to previous policy experiences. The chapter shows how favourable political dynamics and frequent coalition governments formed by the LDS and the SD made it possible to preserve the CPI despite proposals to abolish it (2003, 2011). In the context of the global financial crisis, the lack of institutional veto points and little partisan division in the area of health policy allowed further marketisation measures aimed at securing the financial sustainability of the health sector through increases in co-payments (2012), underlining the path-dependent nature of Slovenian health policy.

Chapter 4 presents the Czech case, detailing how despite a rather difficult start to post-communist health reforms, the country's policymakers demonstrated a remarkable capacity for policy learning. At the same time, moderate political divisions in the context of few institutional constraints generated a protracted learning pattern in which policymakers struggled to integrate further elements of market into policy. The chapter begins by describing the Czech health system under communism, showing how market ideas were triggered by anomalies of the socialist healthcare paradigm. It then shows how the post-communist policymaking setting was marked by relatively soft institutional constraints and a moderate division over health policy between the two major political forces, the Liberal-Conservatives (ODS) and the Social Democrats (ČSSD), shaped by the relationship between the ČSSD and the communist successor party (KSČM). The chapter starts the chronology of health reforms by showing how, in contrast to the Slovenian case, a lack of previous policy experience with healthcare markets under communism contributed to the troubled nature of the first post-communist market reforms (1991, 1992). Even though the reforms led to market failures, in which spiralling costs threw the health system into a crisis, moderate party divides made it possible to adapt market mechanisms (1995, 1996) that substantially stabilised the system. Further episodes of marketisation, including the introduction of deeply controversial user fees for medical services (2007), demonstrate the impact of a moderate party divide and savvy political strategies on overcoming institutional veto points in the policy learning process. Another policy episode, the transformation of public hospitals (1997, 2006, 2011), further highlights the role of the political and institutional contexts in shaping the ongoing struggle to transform Czech healthcare into a market-oriented system.

The last empirical chapter, Chap. 4, shows how the combination of the historical, political, and institutional settings of post-communist health reforms prevented the transformation of market ideas into policy in Poland by generating a disrupted pattern of policy learning over the three post-communist decades. The chapter sets the scene for the Polish case by describing the country's healthcare system under communism, stressing the lack of policy change despite the emergence of market ideas. Moving to the post-communist period, it shows how sharp partisan divisions over health policy were marked initially by conflicts between the unreformed communist successor party (SLD) and the post-Solidarity parties, and subsequently, between the two parties on the right (PO and PiS). The chapter argues a combination of these sharp party divides, unfavourable policy legacies of the health system from communist times, and strong institutional constraints thwarted the process of policy learning. It illustrates this argument by focusing on the key policy episodes, such as the introduction of an insurance system with managed competition, proposed by the post-Solidarity parties (1997, 1998), but then reversed by the SLD (2003). Another major reform effort, the commercialisation of public hospitals (2008, 2011), is another illustration of how continuing party divisions over health policy, now amongst the right-wing block, in combination with institutional constraints activated through both judicial and presidential vetoes, thwarted attempts to marketise Polish healthcare.

Chapter 5 compares health reforms in the three countries, highlighting that despite making similar and parallel efforts to transform market ideas into health policy, Slovenia, the Czech Republic, and Poland followed very different learning paths, thus generating variations in health policy trajectories and reform outcomes. These different paths reflect variation in policy legacies, dynamics of political competition, and institutional settings. To underline how these different learning paths continue to influence policymaking, the chapter briefly compares the healthcare policy in the three countries in the context of the health crisis triggered by the COVID-19 pandemic. The chapter also discusses the main contributions of the book and the policy implications of its main findings. It concludes by suggesting future avenues of research on healthcare reforms in Eastern Europe and beyond.

References

Anderson, Karen M., and Ruud Van Druenen. 2021. The Netherlands. In *Health politics in Europe: A handbook*, ed. E.M. Immergut, K.M. Anderson, C. Devitt, and T. Popic, 520–557. Oxford: Oxford University Press.

Armeanu, Oana I. 2010. *The politics of pension reform in Central and Eastern Europe: Political parties, coalitions, and policies.* New York: Palgrave Macmillan.

Arrow, Kenneth J. 1963. *Uncertainty and the welfare economics of medical care.* Indianapolis: Bobbs-Merrill.

Asensio, Maria. 2021. Portugal. In *Health politics in Europe: A handbook*, ed. E.M. Immergut, K.M. Anderson, C. Devitt, and T. Popic, 275–306. Oxford: Oxford University Press.

Barr, Nicholas A. 2004. *The economics of the welfare state*. Oxford: Oxford University Press.

Bartlett, William, Jadranka Božikov, and Bernd Rechel. 2012. *Health reforms in South-Eastern Europe*. London: Palgrave Macmillan.

Beach, Derek, and Rasmus B. Pedersen. 2013. *Process-tracing methods: Foundations and guidelines*. Ann Arbor: University of Michigan Press.

Bennett, Andrew, and Jeffrey T. Checkel. 2015. Process tracing: From philosophical roots to best practices. In *Process tracing: From metaphor to analytic tool*, ed. Andrew Bennett and Jeffrey T. Checkel, 3–38. Cambridge: Cambridge University Press.

Blomqvist, Paula, and Ulrika Winblad. 2021. Sweden. In *Health politics in Europe: A handbook*, ed. E.M. Immergut, K.M. Anderson, C. Devitt, and T. Popic, 164–204. Oxford: Oxford University Press.

Bohle, Dorothee, and Bela Greskovits. 2012. *Capitalist diversity on Europe's periphery*. Ithaca: Cornell University Press.

Callahan, Daniel, and Anglea Wasunna. 2006. *Medicine and the market: Equity versus choice*. Baltimore: Johns Hopkins University Press.

Chuliá, Elisa. 2021. Spain. In *Health politics in Europe: A handbook*, ed. E.M. Immergut, K.M. Anderson, C. Devitt, and T. Popic, 333–352. Oxford: Oxford University Press.

Cockerham, William C. 2002. *Health and social change in Russia and Eastern Europe*. Abingdon-on-Thames: Routledge.

Della Porta, Donatella, and Michael Keating. 2008. *Approaches and methodologies in the social sciences: A pluralist perspective*. Cambridge and New York: Cambridge University Press.

Elster, Jon, Claus Offe, and Ulrich K. Preuss. 1998. *Institutional design in post-communist societies: Rebuilding the ship at sea*. Cambridge and New York: Cambridge University Press.

Ewert, Benjamin. 2009. Economization and marketization in the German healthcare system: How do users respond? *German Policy Studies* 5 (1): 21–44.

Field, Mark G. 1991. The hybrid profession: Soviet medicine. In *Professions and the state: Expertise and autonomy in the Soviet Union and Eastern Europe*, ed. Anthony Jones. Philadelphia: Temple University.

Ghodsee, Kristen, and Mitchell A. Orenstein. 2021. *Taking stock of shock: Social consequences of the 1989 revolutions*. Oxford: Oxford University Press.

Giaimo, Susan. 2009. *Markets and medicine: The politics of health care reform in Britain, Germany, and the United States*. Ann Arbor: University of Michigan Press.

Gingrich, Jane. 2011. *Making markets in the welfare state: The politics of varying market reforms*. Cambridge and New York: Cambridge University Press.

Gingrich, Jane, and Scott L. Greer. 2021. The United Kingdom. In *Health politics in Europe: A handbook*, ed. E.M. Immergut, K.M. Anderson, C. Devitt, and T. Popic, 115–155. Oxford: Oxford University Press.

Guardiancich, Igor. 2012. *Pension reforms in Central, Eastern and Southeastern Europe: From post-socialist transition to the global financial crisis.* Abingdon-on-Thames: Routledge.

Hayek, Friedrich A. 2007. *The road to serfdom: Text and documents.* Chicago: University of Chicago Press.

Heclo, Hugh. 1974. *Modern social politics in Britain and Sweden: From relief to income maintenance.* New Haven and London: Yale University Press.

Immergut, Ellen M. 1992. *Health politics: Interests and institutions in Western Europe.* Cambridge: Cambridge University Press.

Immergut, Ellen M., and Claus Wendt. 2021. Germany. In *Health politics in Europe: A handbook*, ed. E.M. Immergut, K.M. Anderson, C. Devitt, and T. Popic, 479–519. Oxford: Oxford University Press.

Immergut, Ellen M., Karen M. Anderson, Camilla Devitt, and Tamara Popic. 2021a. *Health politics in Europe: A handbook.* Oxford: Oxford University Press.

Immergut, Ellen M., Diana Burlacu, Andra Roescu, Mirko Wegeman, Tamara Popic, and Guergana Stolarov-Demuth. 2021b. *HEALTHDOX health politics in Europe data set.* EUI Research Data, Department of Political and Social Sciences. https://hdl.handle.net/1814/69838. Accessed 1 July 2022.

Kornai, János. 1992. *The socialist system: The political economy of communism.* Princeton: Princeton University Press.

———. 1997. Reforming the welfare state in postsocialist societies. *World Development* 25 (8): 1183–1186.

Kornai, János, and Karen Eggleston. 2001. *Welfare, choice, and solidarity in transition: Reforming the health section in Eastern Europe.* Cambridge and New York: Cambridge University Press.

Kuitto, Kati. 2016. *Post-communist welfare states in European context: Patterns of welfare policies in Central and Eastern Europe.* Cheltenham and Northampton: Edward Elgar Publishing.

Larsen, Lars T., and Deborah Stone. 2015. Governing health care through free choice: Neoliberal reforms in Denmark and the United States. *Journal of Health Politics, Policy and Law* 40 (5): 941–970.

Le Grand, Julian. 2011. Quasi-market versus state provision of public services: Some ethical considerations. *Public Reason* 3 (2): 80–89.

Le Grand, Julian, and Will Bartlett. 1993. *Quasi-markets and social policy.* Houndmills, Basingstoke: Macmillan Press.

Light, Donald W. 2003. Universal health care: Lessons from the British experience. *American Journal of Public Health* 93 (1): 25–30.

Maino, Franca, and Federico Razetti. 2021. Italy. In *Health politics in Europe: A handbook*, ed. E.M. Immergut, K.M. Anderson, C. Devitt, and T. Popic, 307–332. Oxford: Oxford University Press.

Marrée, Jörgen, and Peter P. Groenewegen. 1997. *Back to Bismarck: Eastern European health care systems in transition*. Aldershot, Hants: Brookfield, Avebury.

Milanovic, Branko. 2014. For whom the wall fell: A balance-sheet of transition to capitalism. *The Globalist*, 7 November. https://www.theglobalist.com/for-whom-the-wall-fell-a-balance-sheet-of-the-transition-to-capitalism. Accessed 10 July 2022.

New York Times. 2008. $1.85 fee to see a doctor? Some say it's too much. https://www.nytimes.com/2008/05/27/world/europe/27czech.html. Accessed 10 July 2022.

Orenstein, Mitchell A. 2008. *Privatizing pensions: The transnational campaign for social security reform*. Princeton and Oxford: Princeton University Press.

Popic, T. 2021. Veto points revisited: The role of party system institutionalization in welfare state change. *Government and Opposition*: 1–22. https://doi.org/10.1017/gov.2021.37.

Ragin, Charles C. 2000. *Fuzzy-set social science*. Chicago: University of Chicago Press.

Rothstein, Bo. 1998. *Just institutions matter: The moral and political logic of the universal welfare state*. Cambridge and New York: Cambridge University Press.

Saltman, Richard B., and Josep Figueras. 1997. *European health care reform: Analysis of current strategies*. Copenhagen: WHO Regional Office for Europe, European Observatory on Health Systems and Policy.

Saltman, Richard B., Reinhard Busse, and Josep Figueras. 2004. *Social health insurance systems in western Europe*. Copenhagen: WHO Regional Office for Europe, European Observatory on Health Systems and Policy.

Schoyen, Mi Ah. 2021. Norway. In *Health politics in Europe: A handbook*, ed. E.M. Immergut, K.M. Anderson, C. Devitt, and T. Popic, 247–270. Oxford: Oxford University Press.

Sokhey, Sarah Wilson. 2017. *The political economy of pension policy reversal in post-communist countries*. Cambridge: Cambridge University Press.

Standing, Guy. 1996. Social protection in Central and Eastern Europe: A tale of slipping anchors and torn safety nets. In *Welfare states in transition: National adaptations in global economies*, ed. G. Esping-Andersen. London: Sage.

Szikra, Dorottya, and Béla Tomka. 2009. Social policy in East Central Europe: Major trends in the twentieth century. In *Post-communist welfare pathways: Theorizing social policy transformations in Central and Eastern Europe*, ed. A. Cerami and P. Vanhuysse. London: Palgrave Macmillan.

Tavits, Margit, and Natalia Letki. 2009. When left is right: Party ideology and policy in post-communist Europe. *American Political Science Review* 103 (4): 555–569.

Thomson, Sarah, Thomas Foubister, and Elias Mossialos. 2009. *Financing health care in the European Union: Challenges and policy responses.* Copenhagen: World Health Organization, European Observatory on Health Systems and Policies.

Toth, Federico. 2021. *Comparative health systems: A new framework.* Cambridge: Cambridge University Press.

Tritter, Johnatan, Meri Koivusalo, Eeva Ollila, and Paul Dorfman. 2009. *Globalisation, markets and healthcare policy: Redrawing the patient as consumer.* Abingdon-on-Thames: Routledge.

Weinerman, E. Richard. 1969. *Social medicine in Eastern Europe: The organization of health services and the education of medical personnel in Czechoslovakia, Hungary, and Poland.* Cambridge: Harvard University Press.

CHAPTER 2

The Politics of Policy Learning

> To become policy, ideas must link up with politics—the mobilization of consent for policy. Politics involves power. Even a good idea cannot become policy if it meets certain kinds of opposition, and a bad idea can become policy if it is able to obtain support. (Gourevitch 1989: 87–88)

Introduction

The previous chapter set the main puzzle of this book, suggesting the development of market-oriented health reforms followed very different paths within three post-communist countries: Slovenia, Czech Republic, and Poland. In Slovenia, this path was marked by *survival*, as the policy introduced in the early transition stood the test of time throughout the three communist decades. The Czech health policy path displayed *instability*, as market elements were introduced but then partially withdrawn. Lastly, in Poland, healthcare policy showed radical *reversals* and failed reform attempts that made the country's health system more closely resemble state-dominated healthcare provision. This book asks why the three countries followed such distinctively different policy paths in the post-communist period.

This chapter develops the central argument of the book by explaining the different paths of post-communist health policy through the conceptual lens of policy *learning*. Learning is defined as a deliberate attempt to adjust policy ideas and adapt them to a specific policymaking context (see

T. Popic, *Health Reforms in Post-Communist Eastern Europe*,
https://doi.org/10.1007/978-3-031-15497-3_2

Hall 1993). Building on the concept of learning understood as adaptation of ideas to policy context, the chapter argues that whilst the post-communist policy reforms in the three countries originated in the departure from the socialist policy paradigm and were driven by the same policy *ideas* of market-oriented healthcare, their policy trajectories varied due to the different policy *learning* experiences. The post-communist healthcare reforms in the three countries originated in market-oriented policy ideas that had already emerged under communism and were based on a normative belief in the superiority of the market over the state in delivering healthcare services. The adoption of these ideas implied a paradigm change in the overall interpretative framework guiding health policy, with a concomitant shift from the state-dominated and public model of health provision to a model in which healthcare is provided through market instruments such as privatisation and competition. Yet as the attempts to translate these ideas into policy took place in markedly different political environments, they met with different levels of success and generated distinctive paths of policy development. The book argues three main contextual factors—policy legacies, political institutions, and party competition—shaped the trial and error dynamics of the health policy learning process differently in Slovenia, Czech Republic, and Poland.

Policy *legacies*—healthcare reforms and policy experiences under communism—influenced the first phase of healthcare policy learning in which policymakers sought to shift to a market-oriented system of healthcare provision in the post-communist context. In Slovenia, policymakers had previously experimented with market-like elements in healthcare and were now more cautious, opting for a gradual approach in introducing the initial market reforms in the post-communist reality. Czech and Polish policymakers lacked a critical view of markets or, indeed, any experience at all with markets as alternatives to state-organised health systems, and they opted for more radical reform. These different approaches had markedly different outcomes—relatively smooth and error-free early reform in Slovenia and textbook examples of market failure in Czech Republic and Poland.

After the initial reforms, the policy developments involved a continued trial and error process shaped by *institutions* and *party competition*. The institutional framework influenced the policymaking by specifying the configurations of veto points that could be used to block reforms based on market ideas. Yet, institutions interacted with the political dynamics in such a way that the effect of these veto points on policy outputs depended on the intensity of party competition (see also Popic 2021a). In Slovenia, light veto arrangements combined with weak party divisions over health policy issues, permitted a relatively smooth learning process that resulted in the *survival* of a limited, but substantially market-oriented, health policy model established in the early transition. Party division over health policy was more intense in Czech Republic, and when this was combined with moderate veto arrangements, the learning process became protracted, ultimately generating an *unstable* policy path marked by continuous back-and-forth of market-oriented reforms. In Poland, the learning process was the most protracted, as institutional configurations generated thick veto arrangements which, in combination with strong party divisions over healthcare issues, led to *reversals* and failed attempts of further marketisation.

The book contributes to two streams of literature on health and policy reform more generally. By explaining the variation in post-communist healthcare policy paths as adaptations of similar policy ideas in different political contexts, it contributes to the study of ideas' role in policy change. Even though ideationally-driven accounts of policy change have been increasing over recent decades, scholars have often stressed the need to account for mechanisms and processes through which ideas exert their influence on policy outputs (Yee 1996; Campbell 2002). Whilst the study of ideas has still met with relative success in the public policy field, it has received meagre attention in the field of comparative politics, even generating scepticism about the role, relevance, and usefulness of ideas as explanatory variables (Checkel et al. 2016). Building on Heclo (1974) and Hall (1993), according to whom policymakers essentially 'puzzle' over policy problems and hence necessarily rely on ideas as cognitive cues to formulate policy solutions, this book argues that market ideas dating back to the communist time were the key drivers of change in the post-communist health policy. Yet, the book also argues that the actual success of these ideas in generating policy change was strongly context-dependent, such that the learning process took place through a trial and error process, that is, not necessarily a process through which ideas incrementally influence policy. In the political arena, an idea's influence on policymaking can be obstructed, reversed, but also bolstered, as shown by the experiences of Czech, Polish, and Slovenian health policy, respectively. In the literature linking ideas and learning, this argument goes beyond the claim that 'ideas matter' in policymaking (see Mehta 2011; Béland et al. 2022) and seeks to explain why in some context they do matter and why in others they do not, in spite of considerable efforts of policymakers. To explain the variation in learning trajectories and understand why some countries are more successful in adopting certain ideas than others, we need to look at politics (Gourevitch 1989), or more specifically, how factors such as policy legacies, institutions, and party competition shape policymakers' attempts to translate these ideas into policy practice.[1]

The book also speaks to the literature on policy feedback (e.g. Pierson 1993; Béland 2010; Jacobs and Weaver 2015). This literature is concerned with mechanisms that account for how policy change influences future policy developments. One branch of policy feedback studies focuses on the role of interests, arguing the adoption of public policies is followed by interest group activities, with interest consolidation a major type of policy feedback (Pierson 1993: 598–599; see also Skocpol 1995). Policy feedback is seen as a self-reinforcing process in which policies strengthen their own political support and expand it over time (Jacobs and Weaver 2015). This book argues that new policies can create favourable conditions for interest group mobilisation. It shows, for example, how policies of privatisation introduced in early transition in Poland, Czech Republic, and Slovenia contributed to the development of professional groups focused on protecting the interests of private health practitioners. Yet as privatisation only led to a fragmentation of interests among wider group of health professionals, the potential of these new interest group formations to actually feed back into policies to strengthen their base was limited. Hence, rather than representing an ongoing consolidation of interests, the key feedback process generated by policy change was the consolidation of ideas, that is, the integration of ideas into the existing policies and institutional set-up of the health system (see Béland 2010). This feedback effect, however, did not always result in the ultimate survival of market ideas in post-communist health policy. As shown in the following comparison of the three countries, the capacity of market-oriented policies to strengthen their support and expand over time was deeply dependent on the political and institutional context, and this made the feedback effect and ideas consolidation in Slovenia easier than in the Czech Republic and Poland.

Lastly, considering ideas as the core element of policy change, the book responds to the call for better conceptualisation of the relationship

[1] Emphasising the definition of learning as process driven by a set of intellectual beliefs (see Blyth 2013) rather than knowledge, this conception departs from the recent literature on policy learning which interprets it as an epistemic process (see Dunlop and Radaelli 2013).

between policy ideas and political power (Béland et al. 2016). Relying on Gourevitch's (1989) claim that ideas have to link with politics in order to influence policy, the book distinguishes between two dimensions of political power: institutional structures and political agency. Whilst its argument underlines the importance of institutional veto points, points in the policymaking process at which reform proposals can be blocked, it understands configurations of these veto points as channels for ideas rather than interests (see Immergut 1990, 1992; Immergut et al. 2021). In addition, the book argues that whether and to what extent ideas can influence policy depends not only on the institutional structures of political power that could potentially constrain the policy process, but also on the context of party competition (see Popic 2021a), more specifically, the extent of cross-party agreement on the main policy goals. In more general terms, this implies that the different paths of ideationally driven policy change, that is, of the policy learning process are the result of the interaction of structure and agency of political power.

The rest of this chapter proceeds as follows. In the first part, it reviews three alternative approaches to the understanding of the variety of the post-communist healthcare policy paths, each of which presents policy outcomes in particular way: as a consequence of *professional power and interests*, as a result of the influence of *external actors*, and as a result of *economic pressures* on the post-communist welfare state. The second part of the chapter provides an elaborate theoretical account of the book's main argument—the politics of policy learning—explaining how each of three factors, *legacies*, *institutions*, and *party competition*, affects the translation of market-oriented ideas into policy, illustrating this argument with examples of health policy episodes from the three countries.

Alternative Explanations

Professional Power

An approach to healthcare policy change based on professional power draws on a distinctive element of the healthcare sector—the medical profession. With origins in the theory of professional dominance (see Johnson 1972), this approach argues the medical profession distinguishes itself from others because it has achieved a position of power based on its monopoly in the healthcare domain. The establishment of this monopoly was enabled by doctors' technical expertise and gradual division of labour through which they gained exclusive rights to autonomy in all spheres of medical practice, as well as exclusive rights to control entry into the profession through medical licencing (Freidson 1970). Once doctors controlled entry to the profession, they could use their monopoly position in the market for healthcare services, and this, in turn, allowed them to corporately control the healthcare sector (Berlant 1975). Their control of the sector placed doctors in a special position from which they could act as a powerful lobby group. The idea that doctors' professional power translates into political power is based on the assumption that the cooperation of policymakers with doctors, as the only professional group officially qualified to carry out medical treatments, is necessary for healthcare reform (see Immergut 1991).

The post-communist period opened up a window of opportunity for a change in the relationship between doctors and the state, as it was a period of professional revival. Under communism, the medical professional went through a process of 'taming', which implied a change from a small, elite, and prestigious profession working in private practice for the rich to a large, publicly employed profession working for the masses (Field 1991). This process of 'taming' was part of the project of medicine 'socialisation', initiated in the early post-war years in Eastern European countries that were under the pervasive influence of the Soviet Union (Weinerman 1969; Field 1991).

Professional healthcare associations were re-established in the post-communist period after almost 40 years of inactivity. The Polish Chamber of Physicians and Dentists (*Naczelna Izba Lekarska*) re-established itself as a professional self-governing body of doctors and dental practitioners in 1989. Similarly, the Czech Chamber of Physicians (*Česká Lekářská Komora*) was re-established in 1991 and the Slovenian Medical Chamber (*Zdravniška Zbornica Slovenije*) in 1992. With the recovery of their legal status, the medical chambers in the three countries quickly achieved an important position within the health sector and took over such tasks as licensing healthcare professionals, enforcing ethical standards of medical practice, and guaranteeing the quality of delivered care. This professional role was strengthened by the introduction of obligatory membership for all practicing physicians, and this, in turn, allowed the chambers to monopolise the interest representation of the medical profession.

Given these trends, it seems reasonable to expect that the post-communist revival of professional medical associations would be matched by a strong professional influence on the policymaking process and its outcomes. Doctors were finally able to organise independently of the state and control the profession from a recognised position of power. Therefore, it could be expected that they would use this newly acquired independence and power as leverage in the policymaking process (see Potůček and Radičová 1997; see also Lawson and Nemec 2003; Roberts 2009; Björkman and Nemec 2013).

However, as the empirical analysis of the three cases in this book will show in more detail, although doctors did try to influence the reform process, the post-socialist revival of the medical profession did not translate into their organised political influence on the policymaking process in any of the three countries. One reason for the lack of professional influence was the fragmentation of interest representation within the medical profession. In spite of obligatory membership, professional interest representation was distorted because the medical profession was divided along different lines. One line of division was retained from socialist times, the division between doctors working in primary and specialist care (Weinerman 1969). Another division emerged as consequence of privatisation, generating conflicts between doctors working in the public and those working in the private sector. New and more explicit divisions were also built on emerging differences in the profitability of particular medical specialties and new approaches to healthcare administration and funding (Healy and McKee 1997; Nelson 2001: 257). Taken together, the multiple divisions led to the emergence of different professional associations, each of which claimed to represent a different professional group and very often expressing opposing demands in the policymaking process (see also Sitek 2010).

In addition, the influence of healthcare professionals on reforms was channelled through political parties. In all three countries, doctors actively took part in the policymaking process as members of government parties and parliamentary health committees and as Ministers of Health. Whilst this generated potential channels of professional influence on healthcare reforms, empirical analysis indicates that doctors did not uniformly support or oppose market reforms, suggesting their policy positions tended to reflect party rather than professional preferences. The primacy of party over professional position is supported by the fact that some of the main market-oriented health reforms proposed by doctors in ministerial positions, such as the introduction of user fees for medical services in the Czech Republic, were strongly opposed by doctors and medical associations more generally. This shows, as argued herein, that the post-communist health policies were not outcomes of doctors' interests but of market ideas and the learning process in which parties and party competition shaped how these ideas were adapted to the specific policy-making context.

External Actors

The approach focusing on the role of external actors in shaping post-communist social policy and, more specifically, health policy reforms rests on an Eastern Europe-specific explanation. According to this view, the transition from socialism to capitalism and democracy created a policy vacuum in post-communist countries, with international organisations, most notably the World Bank, the World Health Organisation, the International Monetary Fund, and, later on, the European Union seizing the opportunity to exert influence by providing financing and policy advice in the welfare sector (Deacon 1993, Deacon and Hulse 1997; Deacon et al. 1997; Kapstein and Milanovic 2001; Cerami 2006; Deacon and Stubbs 2007; Kaasch 2015). The view that the post-communist health policy was influenced by international agencies is inspired by literature on the role these organisations played in guiding the post-communist transition to a market economy (see Deacon et al. 1997). This influence was most famously exhibited though the promotion of the transnational policy paradigm for transition to capitalism, embodied in the Washington Consensus and requiring, amongst other measures, fiscal discipline, deregulation, security of property rights, privatisation, and support of private sector development (Williamson 1990; Stiglitz 2005).

The literature on the influence of international agencies in the post-communist health sector is inconclusive, however. Some studies suggest the impact of external actors on post-communist reform was less profound in healthcare than in other welfare sectors, such as pensions (Nelson 2001; Deacon et al. 1997; Radin 2003, 2008; Cerami 2006). For one thing, there was no blueprint for health reforms (Nelson 2001). In addition, there was a lack of knowledge and internal conflict within these organisations, as well as a conscious choice not to get involved in reforms whose success was not foreseeable (Radin 2003, 2008). Other studies claim that although the international influence was less profound in healthcare than, say, in pensions, external actors, such as the World Bank, did steer the post-communist health reforms, actively advocating specific reforms that were market-oriented and part of their broader neo-liberal approach to welfare policy change in the post-communist context (Müller 1999; Kaasch 2015; Cerami 2006; see also Kaminska et al. 2021).

Empirical studies of the healthcare reforms in Poland, Slovenia, and Czech Republic show that even though international agencies such as the World Bank had no standard blueprint for health reforms, their experts worked closely with the post-communist policymakers and had clear recommendations for the strategy and overall direction of healthcare reforms (World Bank 1990, 1991). Interestingly, however, and in contrast to the prevailing views, these recommendations were significantly less market-oriented then the proposals of the post-communist reformers, as the former advocated retention of some key elements of the communist healthcare system and a very careful introduction of markets and privatisation in the provision of medical services. By stressing the need to preserve some elements of the old system, policy advice expressed the international community's more general worry that post-communist policymakers would be overcome by their enthusiasm and try to eliminate all state elements from the policy framework. They feared, in other words, that the post-communist reformers might 'throw out the baby with the bathwater' (Barr 1994: 290).

In the Czech Republic, for example, the World Bank's experts warned against an unregulated health insurance system, specifically opposing reforms that would imply the introduction of reimbursement schemes, such as fee-for service, because of its tendency to generate pervasive incentives, that is, inducing a demand for healthcare. Similarly, the Bank experts were critical of the Slovenian proposal to increase co-payments for health services, fearing the shifting of healthcare costs onto patients could generate barriers to access for economically vulnerable populations. Yet, these recommendations were disregarded by policymakers.

As this book goes on to show, the reasons for this disregard can be traced to the origins of the post-communist reforms and the impact of socialist legacies on the early reforms. The external actor approach to post-communist welfare reform argues there was a substantial 'policy vacuum' into which external actors stepped with their own reform ideas (see Deacon et al. 1997; Cerami 2006). The book takes exception to this view and argues that instead of being introduced into the post-communist policy debate by external actors, the market-oriented reform ideas had emerged already under communism in response to the crisis of the socialist healthcare sector. They were generated by anomalies of the socialist state-centred, hierarchical policy model and led to a paradigm shift based on normative beliefs that replacing state with market mechanisms would generate more efficient and equitable distribution of healthcare resources. As the book shows, even though external actors tried influencing the reforms of the post-communist health policies, changing these policies involved a process driven by ideas developed in domestic policy circles; that is, they were 'home-grown' and, in some instances, significantly more radical than the reform proposals of external actors.

Economic Pressures

The last explanation argues the main drivers of market-oriented health reform are globalisation and economic pressures. Public policies change under economic pressures generated by globalisation-driven economic integration, a process through which states integrate their economic activity by reducing barriers to movement of labour, trade, and investment. These pressures drive competition between different national systems of government, giving rise to the phenomenon of the 'competition state', whereby the state is primarily concerned with attracting business investment and increasing the competitiveness of its territory (Cerny 1990, 1997; Jessop 2002). The rise of the competition state is seen as having deep consequences for the welfare state. It puts governments under stress, prompting them to opt for specific types of polices that make them more competitive than other countries, such as policies that attract business investment by lowering taxation. This endangers the fiscal basis of the welfare state and, if taken to an extreme, can create a 'race-to-the-bottom', with a downward spiral of social spending cutbacks (Steinmo 1993; Swank 2006; Swank and Steinmo 2002; Genschel 2002). More substantively, the economic pressures and rise of the competition state lead to 'increased marketisation', or the promotion of enterprise and profitability in the public sector and privatisation of services previously provided by the state (Cerny 1997; see also Genschel and Seelkopf 2015).

The argument of economic pressures and the rise of the competition state leading to a race-to-the-bottom of welfare spending and marketisation has been prominent in analyses of post-communist welfare developments (see Vukov 2016). Given the heavy dependence on foreign capital for growth, and as capital cannot be prevented from reallocating to countries where costs of business are lower (i.e. capital flight thesis), governments in these countries are seen as having little option but to accede to the demands of capital for lower taxes and labour costs. This implies that in Eastern Europe, globalisation pressures would be particularly strong, resulting in a shrinking welfare state, with transformations aimed at making the state more competitive by reducing welfare spending and turning to market and private solutions in social policy provision (Kapstein and Milanovic 2001; Cerami and Vanhuysse 2009; Appel and Orenstein 2018).

The approach taken in this book sides with one aspect of the competition state perspective. More specifically, it argues that to understand welfare state developments, we have to look at more substantial transformations of the different roles of the state in the welfare context as these are revealed in the ways state institutions have been trimmed, re-arranged, and re-purposed to provide welfare in modern capitalist democracies (Jessop 2002: 258). Yet in contrast to the competition state theory, the book argues that in the post-communist countries, the market-oriented shift in welfare sectors such as healthcare, which led to the transformation of the state's role in healthcare provision, did not originate in economic but in ideational pressures. The departure from the existing model of healthcare provision (i.e. state domination and central planning) was not a consequence of increasing economic competition but reflective of a paradigm shift in the socialist model of health policy. In Poland, Czech Republic, and Slovenia, the first traces of this paradigm shift appeared under communism, whilst these countries were still relatively isolated from international economic pressures, and was essentially an endogenous process triggered by the crisis of ideas underpinning the socialist healthcare model. This shows that the shift towards markets in healthcare started before these countries turned into capitalist economies and became exposed to global pressures to attract investment and increase competitiveness.

In the post-communist period, health policy was certainly not isolated from the broader context of economic transition. Financial concerns played a role in policy decisions, as shown, for example, in Chap. 3, when the architect of the Polish transition to capitalism, Finance Minister Leszek Balcerowitcz, fought hard to lower health insurance contributions in an attempt to reduce the sector's financial deficit. Yet as shown in the analysis, in all three countries, health reform proposals were generally comprehensive and included substantial, structural transformations of the state's role in healthcare and a shift to markets as instruments of health provision. Implementing these reforms often involved financial risks endangering the stability of the sector as a whole, and in cases of market failure, even led to dramatic increases in healthcare spending, all of which did little to contribute to the competitive state model. This shows that rather than being driven by rationale of economic competitiveness, policy change originated in the cracks of the socialist healthcare paradigm and was essentially an ideationally driven, trial and error process of learning aimed at adapting market ideas into policy.

In what follows, the chapter elaborates on this core argument and explains how the healthcare policy ideas emerging from this paradigmatic shift were shaped by a combination of country-specific policy legacies, party competition, and institutional structures, ultimately creating diverse healthcare policy trajectories across countries.

The Politics of Policy Learning

The book understands policy change as an endogenous process based on learning, with learning defined as 'a deliberate attempt to adjust the goals or techniques of policy in response to past experiences and new information' (Hall 1993: 278). This definition of learning underlines that policymaking is a process in which deliberations about social problems imply new policies as solutions are always constructed as responses to past policy experiences; as such, they represent 'meaningful reactions to previous policies' (Weir and Skocpol 1985: 119). This implies that policy change is not just a replacement of one set of policies with another, but is a cognitive process in which ideas play a central role, and policymaking involves adjustment and adaptation of these ideas to the specific context (Heclo 1974; Hall 1993). Drawing on this key concept of learning, the book maintains that ideas are necessary to trigger policy change and substantially shape its content, building its argument on the so-called ideational turn in public policy analysis—the scholarly shift in attention towards ideas as driving factors of policy change (e.g. Blyth 1997; Campbell 2002; Cox 2004; Béland 2005; Schmidt 2008; Gofas and Hay 2010; Carstensen 2011; Berman 2013).

Whilst the ideational approach to policy change is useful, the book goes beyond it to claim that if we really want to understand why policymaking based on the very same ideas can generate different policy paths and outputs, we have to turn to the study of politics. In the context of the three countries of interest, the health policy legacies of the socialist regime, the institutional setup, and the intensity of party competition over healthcare issues help explain the ideational influence on policy outputs. Hence, the book argues that ideas most certainly matter, but an account of policy change seeking to assess their reach in shaping policy trajectories over time has to consider both the 'puzzling' and the 'powering' parts of the ideational influence on policymaking (see Heclo 1974; Béland et al. 2016).

Figure 2.1 illustrates the analytical framework of policy learning linking ideas with the outputs of the policymaking. This framework breaks down the process of policy learning into two phases—the formulation of policy proposals and the translation of these proposals into policy outputs. As we follow the arrows, we see that whilst ideas and policy paradigms, understood as sets of ideas, act as main drivers of policy reforms, previous policy setups influence policy change, triggering the process whereby new policy proposals emerge as reactions to past policies. This, in turn, sets in motion the process of policy learning; in the initial phase, the incorporation of ideas into policy proposals is shaped by policy legacies, but in the following phase, the translation of these proposals into policy outputs depends on institutions and party competition. Lastly, the arrow from policy outputs to ideas indicates the continuous and cyclical character of policy learning. Once ideas are adapted and translated into policy outputs, policy change takes place, constituting a new policy arrangement. In the subsequent cycle of policy learning, these arrangements act as past policies that influence new policy proposals, whose translation into policy outputs is, again, shaped by institutions and party competition.

The core argument of the book provides new insights that go beyond the dominant views on how legacies, institutions, and political parties influence policymaking. With respect to legacies, the book argues that

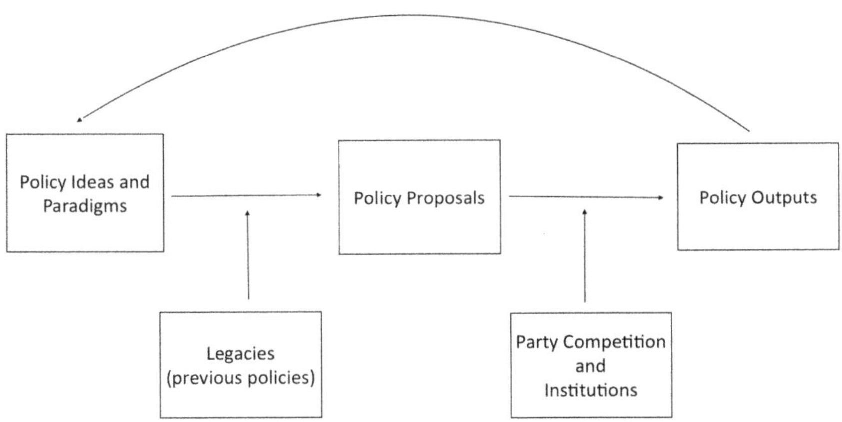

Fig. 2.1 The process of policy learning

health policy change in post-communist Slovenia, Poland, and Czech Republic was not influenced by the legacies of socialism *per se* (see Kornai and Eggleston 2001; Kaminska 2013). Rather, these legacies affected perceptions of available policy options, influencing adaptations of policy ideas to policy context. It also stress the importance of institutions; formally defined rules may specify where in the policymaking process, policy change can be blocked (Immergut 1990; Immergut et al. 2007), but the overall institutional influence on policy change can be properly understood only in the context of party competition. The focus on party competition underlines that it is not the partisanship of the parties in the government that explains the policy change (Tavits and Letki 2009; Careja and Emmenegger 2009). Rather, the relations between the parties—the intensity of party divisions over policy—condition the institutional influence on change and thus influence the policy learning process. If this intensity is low because the main political parties share similar vision of healthcare policy, and if the institutional context features a small number of vetoes, this can enable a learning process marked by a smooth adaptation of ideas into policy outputs and their preservation over time. If these visions are deeply conflictual, and the institutional context is marked by multiple vetoes, the adaptation of policy ideas through the learning process is more difficult, generating a protracted process of policy learning marked by reversals.

This section develops the theoretical framework for the book's core argument in two steps. First, it introduces the concepts of policy paradigms and learning to account for the ideational dimension of health policy change in the post-communist context. Second, it focuses on three specific elements—policy legacies, political institutions, and party competition—outlining how each influenced adaptation and adjustment of market-oriented policy ideas to country-specific policymaking contexts and how this generated a variety of healthcare policy paths across countries.

Ideas, Paradigms, Learning, and Policy Change

The ideational argument of policy change understands policymaking as a process in which its main actors—policymakers—concentrate on seeking solutions for social problems (Heclo 1974; Hall 1993) through a process of 'collective puzzlement on society's behalf' wherein ideas play a central role (Blyth 1997; Berman 1998; Hay 2004; Campbell 2002). The focus on ideas as drivers of policy change emphasises the cognitive nature of policymaking. As they puzzle over social problems, policymakers are guided by a set of ideas containing normative beliefs and values grounded on assumptions reflective of specific world-views, which are taken for granted and lie in the background of the policy debates (Campbell 2002). These normative beliefs define the debates as they constrain the range of choices and alternatives policymakers are likely to perceive as acceptable and legitimate when they formulate new policies. They help policymakers decide which policies are most appropriate, an especially important consideration when there is no conclusive evidence about which policy option is most likely to work best (Campbell 2002).

A core concept in the ideational approach to policy change is the *policy paradigm*. The policy paradigm refers to the 'framework of ideas and standards that specify not only the goals of policy and kind of instruments that can be used to attain them, but also the very nature of the problems they are meant to be addressing' (Hall 1993: 279). As they are based on ideas, policy paradigms constitute a structured intellectual background of policy decisions, which are 'inherently normative and programmatic' and serve as 'road maps' to policymakers by providing a relatively coherent set of assumptions about policy problems and their solutions (Béland 2005: 8).

Even though policy paradigms are normally stable, they can be threatened by the appearance of *anomalies*, unusual developments not fully comprehensible to policymakers, even as puzzles, within the terms of the existing paradigm. As these anomalies accumulate, they gradually undermine the intellectual coherency and precision of the original paradigm, thus leading to its re-consideration. The emergence of a new policy paradigm is triggered by the enduring apparent anomalies in the old paradigm that are leading to policy failures. The movement from one paradigm to another is likely to involve not only the accumulation of anomalies, but also experimentation with new forms of policy and policy failures, precipitating a shift in the locus of authority over policy and initiating a wider political contest between competing paradigms. The new paradigm is accepted if it is considered to have the ability to explain the persistent anomalies more accurately than the set of ideas and standards contained in the old paradigm (Hall 1993).

As hinted earlier in this chapter, market-oriented health policy ideas emerged in response to the failures of socialist healthcare systems employing a state-centred policy paradigm. Shortly after World War II, Poland, Slovakia, and Czech Republic adopted this paradigm as an interpretative framework of healthcare policy based on the normative belief that state instruments, including the centralisation and hierarchisation of healthcare system management, would be the most suitable for reaching the main policy goal—providing good quality, universally accessible medical care to the population. The healthcare systems of the three countries under socialism were not identical in organisational terms, as Slovenia kept its insurance-based system, whilst Poland and the Czech Republic shifted to budget-based financing, but the establishment of the socialist heath paradigm implied strikingly similar policy developments. These involved the elimination of previous instruments of health policy which did not fit the state-centred model, including the private delivery of medical services and the financing of healthcare through patients' payments. Healthcare facilities were nationalised, doctors and healthcare staff became state employees, and a hierarchical, state-dominated model of healthcare financing and provision was established based on strict planning of resource allocation. The socialist health policy based on this paradigm witnessed impressive developments during the early post-war period. The health systems in the three countries significantly increased their coverage which became universal for the first time in the countries' histories and significantly strengthened their healthcare workforce and infrastructure, and this, in turn generated dramatic improvements in the health of their populations.

The first anomalies in the socialist state-centred health policy paradigm emerged in the 1960s and became particularly evident during the 1970s. These anomalies involved shortages of healthcare goods and materials, corruption in the form of patient under-the-table payments to doctors and medical staff, and deterioration in population health. The emergence of anomalies triggered crisis and uncertainty as the socialist policymakers suddenly found themselves facing problems for which the existing paradigm offered no clear-cut solutions (see Campbell 2002; see also Dobbin 1993; Hall 1993; Hay 2004).

The recognition of anomalies and crisis prompted reactions from healthcare professionals and experts who were critical of the existing regime. Criticism also appeared in the official reports of state institutions, including the national institutes for health and healthcare service research. These reactions pointed to the multiple problems facing the socialist healthcare sector and signalled the 'cracks' in the socialist policy paradigm as policymakers traced the main causes of these problems in a policy model based on hierarchical and centralised state-dominated system. In their view, the model generated the wrong incentives for provision of medical care.

Even more importantly, these reactions suggested alternatives to the exclusively state-run system, such as privatisation of care provision or decentralisation of healthcare financing, could offer a way out of the crisis. As indicated in a report written by Czech health policy experts, insufficient financing, shortages of medicines, and corruption were not just 'negative phenomena in healthcare'—as labelled by the authorities. More troublingly, they represented 'a symptom of a disfunctional system' originating in the core principles of the socialist health policy, including its hierarchical character and the state's monopoly on organisation (Charter 77 1984). As such, these views constituted important cognitive steps in the departure from the socialist policy paradigm. They emerged in the context of crisis, characterised by a high degree of uncertainty, and in their questioning of the dominant policy views, they sowed the seeds of ideational change. Advocates of new ideas sought to provide compelling explanations in which old institutions and instruments of policymaking were diagnosed as 'parts of the problem', not as 'parts of the solution' (see Blyth 2002: 5; see also Hay 2004: 207–208).

During late socialism, health systems in all three countries continued to accumulate anomalies, feeding the growing crisis and exacerbating the uncertainty about the future of healthcare. The socialist policymakers suddenly found themselves faced with unusual healthcare problems for which the existing paradigm offered no obvious solutions (see Campbell 2002: 23; see also Hall 1993; Hay 2004). By the end of the 1980s, what was once the core ideal and pride of socialist regimes—easily accessible and good quality healthcare available to the whole population—was a source of shame (see Charter 77 1984). The strong pressure on socialist policymakers to stop the deterioration of the health sector was evident in repeated reform attempts, but also in the open confessions of socialist elites, who were desperately looking for ways out of the crisis. Among the critics, the stubborn appearance of anomalies fed the belief that the application of socialist ideas in healthcare, even in a modified form, was destined to fail, and policymakers needed to find different solutions to resolve the crisis.

Throughout the last socialist decade, in all three countries, healthcare professionals and policy experts continued to criticise the health policy and propose new policy options. In their view, the problems remained unresolved because the guiding principles of health policy remained still confined to the general principles of the socialist policy paradigm, according to which healthcare was provided through a dominantly state-led system of financing and delivery of medical services.[2] Despite the criticism, the health policy of late socialism showed little change. As described by the Polish health policy experts, the period of the 1980s 'witnessed the emergence of very interesting and stimulating concepts and ideas, but was also the period of extreme scarcity of decisions' (Indulski and Włodarczyk 1989: 19). Nevertheless, whilst slow to take hold, the ideas emerging in the criticism were key for subsequent policy change, as they built on the core belief that the market rather than the state-oriented model of healthcare provision was better suited to respond to the population's healthcare needs.

Socialist Health Policy Legacies

The legacy argument, in its most basic form, claims policies introduced under previous policy regimes profoundly influence subsequent policy choices. This legacy argument fits well within the learning framework, according to which previous policy choices influence new policy decisions, contributing to the continuity of policymaking (see Hall 1993). In the literature on the post-socialist restructuring, the legacy argument has also been very influential, with leading scholars concluding that legacies of socialism played a key role in determining the post-socialist pathways (e.g. Offe 1991; Stark and Bruszt 1998; Ekiert and Hanson 2003). One of the more nuanced accounts of the legacies claim in this literature has been that it is not the legacies per se, but rather the experiences and perceptions of these experiences that influenced the post-communist policy choices (see Bohle and Greskovits 2012; Bohle 2017). This understanding of the role of legacies implies that whilst previous policies themselves may not be a matter of choice, the way later policymakers perceive them matters, especially when former policies are complex and controversial and leave ample room for alternative interpretations (Bohle and Greskovits 2012: 66).

The book applies this more nuanced legacy argument to the context of the post-communist health reforms by arguing that the legacies of socialist healthcare influenced the initial post-communist health policy proposals in two ways. One way was through concrete policy *experiences*. As indicated earlier, the three countries had different post-war experiences of health policy, and the crisis in socialist healthcare did not generate the same policy response. Slovenia had a distinctive policy legacy, as after World War II it shifted to the communist model of healthcare provision but kept its

[2] These criticisms were present also in Slovenia, in spite of the shift to the 'soft' version of socialism through introduction of workers' self-management (see Chap. 3).

healthcare insurance system in place. The Slovenian socialist regime was also the most radical in changing policy in the context of crisis. The market socialist reforms under the Josip Broz Tito regime started in the 1970s and led to the development of a specific socialist variant of market reforms based on a unique model of organisation, 'workers' self-management' (Himmelstein et al. 1984; Parmelee 1985; Parmelee et al. 1982). As the workers' self-management model implied substantial decentralisation of the healthcare system and autonomy from the state, it was 'neither market nor state-like' (Parmelee et al. 1982). In contrast, the crisis of the Czech and Polish health policy under socialism did not catalyse significant policy change. These different responses to the socialist health crisis meant the three countries entered the post-socialist period with markedly different baggage of policy experience.

Legacies also influenced how the post-communist policymakers *perceived* the markets in healthcare (see Bohle and Greskovits 2012). As in Slovenia, they had already experimented with alternatives under socialism, their policy experiences were mixed, featuring both a state-run hierarchical policy model and a de-centralised model in which healthcare was provided on the basis of local health needs, so they had a more critical view of the role of state and market in healthcare. On the one hand, they knew the caveats of the state-run health system, including distortions in healthcare provision, such as shortages and corruption. On the other hand, they were aware of policy failures that might occur when healthcare provision departed from the state-run model and was left to local, market-like forces, including lack of coordination, duplication of services, and rising inequalities. These critical views about the role of the state and the market in healthcare strongly influenced the initial health policy choices in post-socialism and were responsible for a 'tailored' approach to market reforms. This included the choice not to privatise healthcare delivery, opting instead to re-centralise the public insurance system and combine it with market elements: patient co-payment for health services and complementary private health insurance.

Czech Republic and Poland inherited different policy legacies that shaped their experiences of organising and managing the health system and their perceptions of the role of market instruments in healthcare provision. The countries had no experience of an organisational structure of healthcare independent of the state, as their post-war governments shifted from an insurance-based healthcare system to the Soviet style, the 'Semashko system' of healthcare, managed exclusively by the central government (Marrée and Groenewegen 1997). Even during the socialist healthcare crisis, Czech and Polish socialist elites remained essentially faithful to the socialist policy model. Thus, their policy legacy was limited to experiences with the state-run model of healthcare provision based on central planning and the hierarchical distribution of available resources. The lack of an encounter with other policy models generated indiscriminate views of alternative, market-oriented healthcare, feeding the perception that only radical market solutions would solve the problems of the health sector. As a result, Czech and Polish policymakers opted for a big-bang approach, introducing large-scale market-oriented reforms, including privatisation of primary care, decentralisation of the insurance system, and establishment of a highly competitive system of healthcare delivery. The differences in legacies hence explain why Slovenian policymakers followed a more selective policymaking style in which they picked from a 'menu' of available market options, whilst Czech and Polish policymakers who lacked a clear understanding of the market's role in healthcare system organisation and had no experience with alternatives to the state-run system went for 'full' reform.

Post-Communist Institutions and Party Competition

The previous section showed how the legacies of socialism shaped the initial choices of health reform; Slovenia took a gradual approach to market reforms, whilst Poland and Czech Republic opted for more radical policy change. Making these different choices involved the adaptation of market ideas to the national healthcare systems shaped by different experiences and perceptions of markets in healthcare—in other words, the countries' respective legacies. Yet, socialist legacies alone cannot explain why the Slovenian healthcare system inaugurated in the 1990s kept its market elements, co-payments, and voluntary insurance and remained unchanged throughout three post-communist decades (*survival*), whilst the Czech trajectory was marked by frequent policy changes (*instability*), and the Polish policy made a U-turn, leading to centralisation and state control and resisting multiple marketisation attempts (*reversal*). These dramatic differences suggest the need to return to the analytical framework of policy learning and look at the other two factors shaping the process—institutions and party competition.

As previously noted, the capacity of institutions to regulate the process of policymaking is conceptualised by the veto points approach (Immergut

1990, 1992). Veto points are 'weak links' in the policymaking process, as they are defined by constitutionally established rules for the various arenas—executive, legislative, electoral, and judiciary—in which government proposals may be blocked (Immergut and Abou-Chadi 2014). As such, veto points are crucial determinants of policy change. The veto points approach emphasises that decisions on a policy proposal are shaped not only by the government, but also by the opposition who can block the proposal in the parliament through a presidential veto, question it in a referendum, or demand checks on its constitutionality in the constitutional court. Each of these points is based on a constitutional rule that grants the power of veto to an actor or to a group of actors in the political system, and this, in turn, enables them to block a departure from the status quo. The opposition to reform who has access to these points in the political decision-making process can block a government proposal for policy change, thus implying the fate of the proposal will substantially depend on the distribution of veto points established by the constitutional rules (see Immergut 1990).

The advantage of using the veto points approach to analyse policy learning is that it views policymaking as a sequential process comprising a series of decisions in different policy arenas, made at different points in time and by different actors. Introducing new policies hence implies a chain of decisions which can be blocked through veto points at various links of the chain. Policy decisions thus require agreement at several points, and the fate of proposals for change depends on the number and location of opportunities for disagreement (see Immergut 1992: 27–28). Institutions as formal rules of policymaking define not only how many veto points are along the decision-making chain, but also who can steer the policymaking process and when those steering it can block departure from the status quo. As such, veto points constitute crucial institutional elements that influence the translation of policy proposals into policy outputs.

The constitutional arrangements in the three countries generated different configurations of institutional veto points: *light* in Slovenia, *medium* in the Czech Republic, and *thick* in Poland (Table 2.1). The 1991 Slovenian Constitution set up a relatively *light* configuration of vetoes characterised by a weakly bicameral Parliament in which the National Assembly (*Državni Zbor*) as the Lower House was given rights to prepare and pass bills with a majority of votes, whilst the Upper House, the National Council (*Državni Svet*), was vested with relatively weak veto

Table 2.1 Veto points configurations in Slovenia, Czech Republic, and Poland

	Parliament	*President*	*Judiciary*	*Referendum*
Slovenia (light)	Weak bicameralism	No veto powers	Constitutional review, binding	Electoral review, binding
Czech Republic (medium)	Moderate bicameralism	Moderate veto powers	Constitutional review, binding	Electoral review, binding
Poland (thick)	Moderate bicameralism	Strong veto powers	Constitutional review, binding	Electoral review, binding

Source: Author's compilation

powers over the policy process. More specifically, its veto of bills passed in the Assembly was defined as conditional on the support of the absolute majority of the Assembly's votes and restrictive, since the Assembly was given power to veto only an entire law, not its parts, and this power of veto was also subject to time limits.[3] The Constitution also gave no rights of veto to the President, but allowed bills or laws to be questioned through Constitutional Court or by public referendum and qualified the decisions made in the judicial and electoral arena as binding (Constitution of the Republic of Slovenia 1991). In contrast, the 1992 Czech Constitution introduced veto configurations of a *medium* strength, drawing on a moderate bicameralism in which the Senate (*Senát*) as the Upper House, with no restrictions, was able to veto decisions by the Lower House, the Chamber of Deputies (*Poslanecká Sněmovna*), even though this veto could be overturned by the absolute majority of votes in the latter. The Constitution also granted the President veto powers, but these were also relatively moderate, as the President's veto depended on the support of the majority of votes in the Chamber. The Constitutional Court and the electorate also had veto powers (Constitution of the Czech Republic 1992). Lastly, Poland's veto configurations defined by the 1997 Constitution were *thick*. The Parliament featured a relatively moderate bicameral structure in which the Senate (*Senate*) as the Upper House could veto the law and the Lower House, the Sejm (*Sejm*), needed the absolute majority of votes to overrule the veto of the Senate. However, In stark contrast to the Slovenian and Czech Constitutions, the Polish Constitution

[3] For further explanation of weak bicameralism in Slovenia, see Chap. 3, *Institutions: Light Veto Points Configurations*.

specified strong veto powers for the President, establishing that the Sejm would need more than three fifths of its votes to overturn a presidential veto.[4] The Polish Constitution also established judicial and electoral vetoes through the Constitutional Court and a referendum (Constitution of the Republic of Poland 1997).

These different veto configurations played a key role in shaping the process of policy learning through which policymakers tried to turn their market-oriented policy proposals into actual policies. In all three countries, Constitutional Courts and electorates constituted veto arenas, as policy proposals could be subject to constitutional and electoral review. What differed was the relative power assigned to the different houses of Parliament and the President. The Slovenian veto configuration made the Lower House the only veto arena in which government proposals for policy change could be blocked. In the Czech Republic, moderate bicameralism made the passage of the policy proposals passed in the Lower House dependent on the lack of vetoes by the Upper House and the President, even though when these vetoes occurred, they could be overturned by majorities in the Lower House. In Poland, besides similarly moderate bicameralism, the President's veto which required larger majority to be overturned in the Lower House was an additional and most serious threat to reform.

Even though these veto configurations constituted formal 'blockages' of the policymaking process, looking at these rules alone cannot account for the institutional influence on policy learning. Indeed, previous studies have recognised that constitutional rules define *ex-ante* where in the policymaking procedure there is a possibility of veto, but they do not define who or more specifically what kind of actors populate these locations. This essentially depends on the political arrangements established through party competition and elections (Immergut 1990, 1992; Immergut and Abou-Chadi 2014). Results of electoral competition which *ex-post* define political actors populating the different arenas matter as much as formal constitutional rules that define the positions of the veto points in the policymaking process. This tight link between veto points and political arrangements emphasises that these points represent points of strategic uncertainty at which policy change can be thwarted. In fact, even a small

[4] The initial constitutional provision set two thirds (2/3) (66.66 per cent) of the votes in the Lower House as required for a President's veto to be overturned, which changed into three fifths (3/5) (60 per cent) of votes in 1997 (Popic 2021b).

shift in electoral results may change the location and strategic importance of a veto point. Thus, institutional configurations and political arrangements—including both constitutional rules and a particular distribution of political actors—define the environment of policymaking (Immergut 1990).

The usual approach to the role of political arrangements in shaping policy change is to focus on *partisanship*. By concentrating on political parties as the main actors in the policy arena, the partisanship approach suggests party ideologies will be particularly important for policy outputs (Iversen and Cusack 2000; Huber and Stephens 2001). Healthcare reforms are often seen by political parties as unique opportunities to express their distinctive ideological profiles and are often used to gain partisan votes (Immergut 1992). More specifically, partisanship theory would assume health policy choices can be attributed, in large part, to the party composition and the ideological profile of the government. According to the traditional left–right division, governments dominated by parties of the left are expected to favour state control of the health sector, whilst governments dominated by the right will prefer minimised state intervention and the introduction of market-like mechanisms in healthcare provision, including privatisation and competition (see Bellido et al. 2019; Potrafke 2017).

The literature on the influence of partisanship on post-communist health policy has yielded inconclusive findings. One is that whilst partisanship matters for social and health spending, its effect on policy outputs in Eastern Europe has been the opposite to that of the West, as Eastern European parties on the left opted for cuts in healthcare spending, and parties on the right followed expansion (Tavits and Letki 2009). Other studies have questioned this relationship between partisanship and social policy outputs, finding partisanship in Eastern Europe matters in a traditional way, with right-wing conservative parties following policies of fiscal retrenchment in the healthcare sector and left-wing parties opting for generous healthcare arrangements (Beckmann et al. 2020; see also Careja and Emmenegger 2009). Yet other studies suggest partisanship does not matter for post-communist social and, more specifically, healthcare spending (Appel and Orenstein 2018; Coman 2019).

As this book goes on to show, the traditional left–right distinction provides little help in capturing the differential influence of parties on post-communist health policies. Instead, to understand how party politics shaped the process of health policy learning, we need to look at the country-specific *intensity of party division* over health issues. Slovenia,

Czech Republic, and Poland displayed different intensities: *weak* in Slovenia, *moderate* in Czech Republic, and *strong* in Poland. In Slovenia, the *weak* intensity of divisions over health issues characteristic of the first decade and a half of post-communism was a result of policy agreement between the parties (LDS and ZLSD/SD), who dominated the country's transition from communism. In Czech Republic, the *moderate* intensity of party divide was marked by a more traditional division between the right (ODS) and the social democratic left (ČSSD). In Poland, the *strong* intensity of party divisions was initially the result of a policy disagreement between the right (e.g. UW, AWS) and the left (SLD), but during the second transitional decade, this conflict was replaced by a conflict between the two parties on the right (PO and PiS).

These different patterns of party competition did not always follow a traditional left–right divide and can be explained by the differences in a specific feature of the post-communist party systems of the three countries—the transformation, identity, and political success of the left parties, in particular, the communist successor parties. Given the countries' socialist past, the parties on the left of the political spectrum in Eastern Europe were mainly represented by communist successor parties (see Ishiyama 1995, 2001; Kostelecký 2002; Grzymała-Busse 2002). After the fall of communism, these parties had to make choices—first, whether to remain on the political scene and second, if they remained as the communist successor parties, whether to transform themselves or retain their orthodox socialist views (see Grzymała-Busse 2002). Despite this commonality, the programmatic transformation of the formerly ruling parties was very country-specific. Their electoral success or failure differed across countries and depended on the extent to which they were able to adapt their strategies and tactics to the changing political environment (see Ishiyama and Bozóki 2001; Grzymała-Busse 2002). The result was a variety of parties on the left, a unique feature of the post-communist party systems (see Ziblatt 1998).

In fact, the main left-wing parties in the three countries had different identities that varied depending on their links to the communist past and subsequent transformation or lack thereof. These identities were important as they affected their readiness to accept or resist market reforms in health, and this, in turn, generated different intensities of party competition over health policy. The Slovenian communist successor party (ZLSD) successfully transformed from a communist party to a party supportive of market-oriented solutions to public policy problems. This transformation was important for ZLSD's identity, as it understood the need to depart from its socialist past to become a social-democratic party and take part in post-communist power arrangements (see Cabada 2005). Even through it could be its main opponent, the ZLSD often formed a coalition with LDS (Fink-Hafner 2006), the centrist-left party leading the Slovenian transition to capitalism and the main advocate of markets in health, and supported LDS's market-oriented reforms, such the establishment of voluntary private health insurance. This resulted in the lack of a significant party divide on health issues; thus, the Slovenian post-communist health politics saw a significant degree of *consensus* on health policy goals; this, in turn, allowed smooth policy learning and relatively easy integration of the market elements into healthcare provision.

In contrast, the identity of the strongest left party in Czech Republic (ČSSD) was marked by the party's pre-communist social-democratic roots. The party claimed it was a 'genuine' left party, with roots in the inter-war period; as such, it could easily be dissociated from socialism (Mansfeldová 2013). It focused on building an identity different from its main competitor on the left side of the political spectrum—the unreformed communist successor party (KSČM)—by insisting on its social democratic origins and frequently adopting Western style 'third way' policies. Rather than working with KSČM, ČSSD was ready to forge political *compromises* with ODS, a right-wing party and the main advocate of market reforms in health. Whilst ČSSD opposed the radical market reforms, they were willing to accept and contribute to the adaptation of the market elements promoted by ODS, such as decentralisation, limited competition, user fees, and consumer-oriented patients' rights.

Lastly, in Poland the main opponent of market reforms was the only partially transformed communist successor party (SLD). The SLD stands out in the region as it was electorally the most successful communist successor party in the Eastern Bloc (Grzymała-Busse 2002). Even though in other welfare policy areas such as pensions, SLD consistently supported pro-market reforms (see Ishiyama and Shafqat 2000; Guardiancich 2012), in health, the party views wavered between the socialist principles of universal, free, and centrally provided healthcare dominated by the state on the one hand and a market-led health sector on the other. Most importantly for health policy development, the SLD was responsible for a radical reversal of market reforms in 2003, marking a policy U-turn characterised by re-centralisation and the return of the state. The Polish pattern of party competition also differed from the competition in the other two countries in that the disappearance of SLD from the Poland's political landscape in the mid-2000s was followed by the emergence of a new *conflict* over health policy between two right parties, the liberal PO and the conservative PiS. As this new pattern of political competition involved policy disagreement between the two right-wing parties, it transcended the traditional partisan division into left and right.

As stressed earlier, the party competition dynamic works together with the veto configurations to create a unique policymaking environment. To be precise, a country-specific combination of political party divisions, or lack thereof, over healthcare and institutional setups with different policy constraints shaped the process of policy learning and the integration of market-oriented elements in healthcare provision in Slovenia, Poland, and Czech Republic (Table 2.2).

In Slovenia, a combination of light veto configuration and weak party divisions allowed a relatively easy *survival* of a country-specific model of health policy strongly reliant on market elements of voluntary private healthcare insurance. This meant that after the successful initial adaptation of market ideas thanks to previous policy experiences, the combination of institution and politics permitted a continued, smooth learning process over time, allowing policymakers to work on further incorporation of market ideas into policy; consequently, voluntary health insurance became an integral part of the health system. In contrast, in the Czech Republic, a combination of a more constraining veto configuration and moderate party division over health issues generated a context in which the learning process was more protracted, making enactment of market reforms into policy more difficult. This led to an *unstable* pattern of policy developments. Lastly, in Poland, thick veto configurations, in combination with very divisive party positions over health issues, made the adaptation of

Table 2.2 Veto points, party divisions over health policy, and trajectories of market-oriented health policy in Slovenia, Czech Republic, and Poland

Veto points		**Party divisions**		
		Weak	**Moderate**	**Strong**
	Light	Slovenia (survival)		
	Medium		Czech Republic (instability)	
	Thick			Poland (reversal)

market ideas into policy particularly strenuous. Conflicting parties' disagreements on healthcare policy goals and multiple institutional opportunities to obstruct market reforms resulted in policy *reversals*, preventing the formulation of successful strategies to adapt market ideas to the Polish health system.

Conclusion

This chapter presents the main argument of the book. It claims that post-communist healthcare reforms originated in the market ideas emerging when the state-socialist paradigm of healthcare provision fell apart. Whilst the ideas driving post-communist health reforms were substantially similar in Poland, Slovenia, and Czech Republic, their influence on policy was not so straightforward. Instead, we see a policy learning process wherein these ideas, through trial and error, were adapted to the policymaking context. These adaptations were shaped by different legacies, institutional structures, and political dynamics. The chapter substantiates the book's key theoretical claims, pointing to the differences in healthcare policy choices and explaining trajectories across countries. The next chapters provide more elaborate empirical support of the core argument via in-depth descriptions of how legacies, institutions, and party competition shaped the adaptation of market ideas to the Slovenian, Czech, and Polish healthcare systems.

References

Appel, Hilary and Orenstein, Mitchell A. 2018. *From triumph to crisis: Neoliberal economic reform in postcommunist countries.* Cambridge University Press.

Barr, Nicholas A. 1994. *Labor markets and social policy in Central and Eastern Europe: The transition and beyond.* Washington, DC: World Bank Publications.

Beckmann, Joscha, Reiner Schweickert, Markus Ahlborn, and Inna Melnykovska. 2020. Drivers of government activity in European countries: Do partisan politics still divide East and West? *Journal of Common Market Studies* 58 (5): 1235–1251.

Béland, Daniel. 2005. Ideas and social policy: An institutionalist perspective. *Social Policy & Administration* 39 (1): 1–18.

———. 2010. The idea of power and the role of ideas. *Political Studies Review* 8 (2): 145–154.

Béland, D., Martin B. Carstensen, and Leonard Seabrooke. 2016. Ideas, political power and public policy. *Journal of European Public Policy* 23 (3): 315–317.

Béland, Daniel, Gregory P. Marchildon, Michele Mioni, and Klaus Petersen. 2022. Translating social policy ideas: The Beveridge report, transnational diffusion, and post-war welfare state development in Canada, Denmark, and France. *Social Policy & Administration* 56 (2): 315–328.

Bellido, Héctor, Lorena Olmos, and Juan Antonio Román-Aso. 2019. Do political factors influence public health expenditures? Evidence pre-and post-great recession. *The European Journal of Health Economics* 20 (3): 455–474.

Berlant, Jeffrey L. 1975. *Profession and monopoly: A study of medicine in the United States and Great Britain*. Berkeley: University of California Press.

Berman, Sheri. 1998. *The social democratic moment: Ideas and politics in the making of interwar Europe*. Cambridge: Harvard University Press.

———. 2013. Ideational theorizing in the social sciences since policy paradigms, social learning, and the state. *Governance* 26 (2): 217–237.

Björkman, James W., and Juraj Nemec. 2013. *Health reforms in Central and Eastern Europe*. The Netherlands: Eleven International Publishing.

Blyth, Mark. 1997. Any more bright ideas? The ideational turn of comparative political economy. *Comparative Politics* 29 (2): 229–250.

———. 2002. *Great transformations: Economic ideas and institutional change in the twentieth century*. Cambridge: Cambridge University Press.

———. 2013. *Austerity: The history of a dangerous idea*. Oxford: Oxford University Press.

Bohle, Dorothee. 2017. Varieties of capitalism in Eastern Europe. In *The Routledge handbook of East European politics*, ed. A. Fagan and P. Kopecký, 267–280. Abingdon-on-Thames: Routledge.

Bohle, Dorothee, and Bela Greskovits. 2012. *Capitalist diversity on Europe's periphery*. Ithaca: Cornell University Press.

Cabada, Ladislav. 2005. Slovenian United list of social democrats: Post-communist or/and post-modern political party? In *Trajectories of the left social democratic and (ex) communist parties in contemporary Europe: Between past and future*, ed. L. Kopeček, 150–164. Brno: Masaryk University, Democracy and Culture Studies Centre.

Campbell, John L. 2002. Ideas, politics, and public policy. *Annual Review of Sociology* 28 (1): 21–38.

Careja, Romana, and Patrick Emmenegger. 2009. The politics of public spending in post-communist countries. *East European Politics and Societies* 23 (2): 165–184.

Carstensen, Martin B. 2011. Ideas are not as stable as political scientists want them to be: A theory of incremental ideational change. *Political Studies* 59 (3): 596–615.

Cerami, Alfio. 2006. *Social policy in Central and Eastern Europe: The emergence of a new European welfare regime*. Münster: LIT Verlag.

Cerami, Alfio, and Pieter Vanhuysse. 2009. *Post-communist welfare pathways: Theorizing social policy transformations in Central and Eastern Europe*. London: Palgrave Macmillan.

Cerny, Philip G. 1990. *The changing architecture of politics: Structure, agency and the future of the state*. London: Sage Publications.

———. 1997. Paradoxes of the competition state: The dynamics of political globalization. *Government and Opposition* 32 (2): 251–274.

Charter 77. 1984. Zdraví je současti práva na život. Praha, Charta 77, dok. č.14/84 z 15. srpna 1984. Listy, Časopis ceskoslovenské socialistické opozice, Príloha k č. 6, 1984. http://scriptum.cz/soubory//scriptum/listyrim/listy_1984_6_priloha_zm_ocr.pdf. Accessed 10 March 2022.

Checkel, Jeffrey, Jeffrey Friedman, Matthias Matthijs, and Roger Smith. 2016. Roundtable on ideational turns in the four subdisciplines of political science. *Critical Review* 28 (2): 171–202.

Coman, Emanuel E. 2019. When left or right do not matter: Ideology and spending in Central and Eastern Europe. *Research & Politics* 6 (1): 1–19.

Constitution of the Czech Republic. 1992. https://www.psp.cz/en/docs/laws/1993/1.html. Accessed 5 March 2022.

Constitution of the Republic of Poland. 1997. https://www.constituteproject.org/constitution/Poland_1997.pdf. Accessed 23 December 2021.

Constitution of the Republic of Slovenia. 1991. http://www.us-rs.si/legal-basis/constitution/?lang=en. Accessed 2 June 2021.

Cox, Robert. 2004. The path-dependency of an idea: Why Scandinavian welfare states remain distinct. *Social Policy & Administration* 38 (2): 204–219.

Deacon, Bob. 1993. Developments in East European social policy. In *New perspectives on the welfare state in Europe*, ed. C. Jones, 177–197. London: Routledge.

Deacon, Bob and Hulse, Michelle 1997. The making of post-communist social policy: The role of international agencies. *Journal of Social Policy*, 26(1): 43–62.

Deacon, Bob, and Paul Stubbs. 2007. *Social policy and international interventions in South East Europe*. Cheltenham: Edward Elgar Publishing.

Dobbin, Frank R. 1993. The social construction of the great depression: industrial policy during the 1930s in the United States, Britain, and France. *Theory and Society* 22(1): 1–56.

Dunlop, Claire A., and Claudio M. Radaelli. 2013. Systematising policy learning: From monolith to dimensions. *Political Studies* 61 (3): 599–619.

Ekiert, Grzegorz, and Stephen E. Hanson. 2003. *Capitalism and democracy in Central and Eastern Europe: Assessing the legacy of communist rule*. Cambridge: Cambridge University Press.

Field, Mark. 1991. The hybrid profession: Soviet medicine. In *Professions and the state: Expertise and autonomy in the Soviet Union and Eastern Europe*, ed. Anthony Jones, 43–62. Philadelphia: Temple University.

Fink-Hafner, Danica. 2006. Slovenia: Between bipolarity and broad coalition-building. In *Post-communist EU member states: Parties and party systems*, ed. S. Jungerstam-Mulders, 217–246. London: Routledge.

Freidson, Eliot. 1970. *Profession of medicine: A study of the sociology of applied knowledge*. New York: Dodd, Mead.

Genschel, Phillip. 2002. Globalization, tax competition, and the welfare state. *Politics & Society* 30 (2): 245–275.

Genschel, Phillip, and Laura Seelkopf. 2015. The competition state. In *The Oxford handbook of transformations of the state*, ed. Stephan Leibfried, Evelyne Huber, Matthew Lange, Jonah D. Levy, Frank Nullmeier, and John D. Stephens, 237–252. Oxford: Oxford University Press.

Gofas, Andreas, and Colin Hay. 2010. The ideational turn and the persistence of perennial dualisms. In *The role of ideas in political analysis: A portrait of contemporary debates*, ed. A. Gofas and C. Hay. New York: Routledge.

Gourevitch, Peter. 1989. Keynesian politics: The political sources of economic policy choices. In *The political power of economic ideas: Keynesianism across nations*, ed. P. Hall. Princeton: Princeton University Press.

Grzymała-Busse, Anna M. 2002. *Redeeming the communist past: The regeneration of communist parties in East Central Europe*. Cambridge: Cambridge University Press.

Guardiancich, Igor 2012. *Pension reforms in Central, Eastern and Southeastern Europe: From post-socialist transition to the global financial crisis*. Abingdon-on-Thames: Routledge.

Hall, Peter A. 1993. Policy paradigms, social learning, and the state: The case of economic policymaking in Britain. *Comparative Politics* 25 (3): 275–296.

Hay, Colin. 2004. Ideas, interests and institutions in the comparative political economy of great transformations. *Review of International Political Economy* 11 (1): 204–226.

Healy, Judith, and Martin McKee. 1997. Health sector reform in Central and Eastern Europe: The professional dimension. *Health Policy and Planning* 12 (4): 286–295.

Heclo, Hugh. 1974. *Modern social politics in Britain and Sweden: From relief to income maintenance*. New Haven: Yale University Press.

Himmelstein, David U., Slobodan Lang, and Steffi Woolhandler. 1984. The Yugoslav health system: Public ownership and local control. *Journal of Public Health Policy* 5 (3): 423–431.

Huber, Evelyn, and John D. Stephens. 2001. Welfare state and production regimes in the era of retrenchment. In *The new politics of the welfare state*, ed. P. Pierson, 107–145. Oxford: Oxford University Press.

Immergut, Ellen M. 1990. Institutions, veto points, and policy results: A comparative analysis of health care. *Journal of Public Policy* 10 (4): 391–416.

———. 1991. Medical markets and professional power: The economic and political logic of government health programs (Vol. 24). Centro de Estudios Avanzados en Ciencias Sociales, Instituto Juan March de Estudios e Investigaciones.

———. 1992. *Health politics: Interests and institutions in Western Europe*. Cambridge: Cambridge University Press.

Immergut, Ellen M., and Tarik Abou-Chadi. 2014. How electoral vulnerability affects pension politics: Introducing a concept, measure and empirical application. *European Journal of Political Research* 53 (2): 269–287.

Immergut, Ellen M., Karen M. Anderson, and Isabel Schulze. 2007. *The handbook of West European pension politics*. Oxford: Oxford University Press.

Immergut, Ellen M., Karen M. Anderson, Camilla Devitt, and Tamara Popic. 2021. *Health politics in Europe: A handbook*. Oxford: Oxford University Press.

Indulski, Jan, and W. Cezary Włodarczyk. 1989. Projects of health system reform in Poland. Paper presented at the seminar *Changing health care systems: Situation and perspective*, Kiel, 23–24 May.

Ishiyama, John. 1995. Communist parties in transition: Structures, leaders, and process of democratization in Eastern Europe. *Comparative Politics* 27 (2): 147–166.

———. 2001. Sickles into roses: The successor parties and democratic consolidation in post-communist politics. In *Party development and democratic change in post-communist Europe*, ed. P. Lewis. Abingdon-on-Thames: Routledge.

Ishiyama, John, and Andras Bozóki. 2001. Adaptation and change: Characterizing the survival strategies of the communist successor parties. *The Journal of Communist Studies and Transition Politics* 17 (3): 32–51.

Ishiyama, John T., and Sahar Shafqat. 2000. Party identity change in post-communist politics: The cases of the successor parties in Hungary, Poland and Russia. *Communist and Post-Communist Studies* 33 (4): 439–455.

Jacobs, Alan M. and Weaver, Kent R. 2015. When policies undo themselves: Self-undermining feedback as asource of policy change. *Governance*, 28(4): 441–457.

Iversen, Torben, and Thomas R. Cusack. 2000. The causes of welfare state expansion: Deindustrialization or globalization? *World Politics* 52 (3): 313–349.

Jessop, Bob. 2002. *The future of the capitalist state*. Cambridge: Polity.

Johnson, Terence J. 1972. *Professions and power*. London: Macmillan.

Kaasch, Alexandra. 2015. *Shaping global health policy: Global social policy actors and ideas about health care systems*. London: Palgrave Macmillan.

Kaminska, Monika E. 2013. The missing dimension: A comparative analysis of healthcare governance in Central and Eastern Europe. *Journal of Comparative Policy Analysis: Research and Practice* 15 (1): 68–86.

Kaminska, Monika E., Ertila Druga, Liva Stupele, and Ante Malinar. 2021. Changing the healthcare financing paradigm: Domestic actors and international organizations in the agenda setting for diffusion of social health insurance in post-communist Central and Eastern Europe. *Social Policy & Administration* 55 (6): 1066–1081.

Kapstein, Ethan B., and Branko Milanovic. 2001. Responding to globalization. Social policy in emerging market economies. *Global Social Policy* 1 (2): 191–212.

Kornai, János, and Karen Eggleston. 2001. *Welfare, choice and solidarity in transition: Reforming the health sector in Eastern Europe*. Cambridge: Cambridge University Press.

Kostelecký, Tomáš. 2002. *Political parties after communism: Developments in East-Central Europe*. Washington, DC: Woodrow Wilson Center Press.

Lawson, Colin, and Juraj Nemec. 2003. The political economy of Slovak and Czech health policy: 1989–2000. *International Political Science Review* 24 (2): 219–235.

Mansfeldová, Zdenka. 2013. The Czech Republic. In *The handbook of political change in Eastern Europe*, ed. S. Berglund, 217–253. Cheltenham: Edward Elgar Publishing.

Marrée, Jörgen, and Peter P. Groenewegen. 1997. *Back to Bismarck: Eastern Europe health care systems in transition*. Avebury: Ashgate.

Mehta, Jal. 2011. The varied roles of ideas in politics: From whether to how. In *Ideas and politics in social science research*, ed. D. Béland and R.H. Cox, 23–26. New York: Oxford University Press.

Müller, Katharina. 1999. *The political economy of pension reform in Central and Eastern Europe*. Cheltenham and Northampton: Edward Elgar.

Nelson, Joan. 2001. The politics of pension and healthcare reform in Hungary and Poland. In *Reforming the state: Fiscal and welfare reform in post-socialist countries*, ed. J. Kornai, S. Haggard, and R.R. Kaufman, 235–266. Cambridge: Cambridge University Press.

Offe, Claus. 1991. Capitalism by democratic design? Democratic theory facing the triple transition in East Central Europe. *Social Research* 58 (2): 865–892.

Parmelee, Donna E. 1985. Whither the state in Yugoslav Health Care? *Social Science & Medicine* 21 (7): 719–728.

Parmelee, Donna E., Gail Henderson, and Myron Cohen. 1982. Medicine under socialism: Some observations on Yugoslavia and China. *Social Science & Medicine* 16 (15): 1389–1396.

Pierson, Paul 1993. When effect becomes cause: Policy feedback and political change. *World Politics*, 45(4): 595–628.

Popic, Tamara. 2021a. Veto points revisited: The role of party system institutionalization in welfare state change. *Government and Opposition*: 1–22. https://doi.org/10.1017/gov.2021.37.

———. 2021b. Poland. In *Health politics in Europe: A handbook*, ed. E.M. Immergut, K.M. Anderson, C. Devitt, and T.Popic, 745–766. Oxford: Oxford University Press.

Potrafke, Niklas. 2017. Partisan politics: The empirical evidence from OECD panel studies. *Journal of Comparative Economics* 45 (4): 712–750.

Potůček, Martin, and Iveta Radičová. 1997. Splitting the welfare state: The Czech and Slovak cases. *Social Research* 64 (4): 1549–1587.

Radin, Dagmar. 2003. The impact of the World Bank on health care reform in transitional economies. *Politička Misao* 40 (5): 30–51.

———. 2008. World Bank funding and health care sector performance in Central and Eastern Europe. *International Political Science Review* 29 (3): 325–347.

Roberts, Andrew. 2009. The politics of healthcare reform in postcommunist Europe: The importance of access. *Journal of Public Policy* 29 (3): 305–325.

Schmidt, Vivien A. 2008. Discursive institutionalism: The explanatory power of ideas and discourse. *Annual Review of Political Science* 11: 303–326.

Sitek, Michał. 2010. The new institutionalist approaches to health care reform: Lessons from reform experiences in Central Europe. *Journal of Health Politics, Policy and Law* 35 (4): 569–593.

Skocpol, Theda 1995. *Protecting soldiers and mothers: The political origins of social policy in the United States*. Harvard University Press.

Stark, David, and Laszlo Bruszt. 1998. *Postsocialist pathways: Transforming politics and property in East Central Europe*. Cambridge: Cambridge University Press.

Steinmo, Sven. 1993. *Taxation and democracy: Swedish, British, and American approaches to financing the modern state*. New Haven: Yale University Press.

Stiglitz, Joseph E. 2005. More instruments and broader goals: Moving toward the post-Washington consensus. In *Wider perspectives on global development*, 16–48. London: Palgrave Macmillan.

Swank, Duane. 2006. Tax policy in an era of internationalization: Explaining the spread of neoliberalism. *International Organization* 60 (4): 847–882.

Swank, Duane, and Sven Steinmo. 2002. The new political economy of taxation in advanced capitalist democracies. *American Journal of Political Science* 46 (3): 642–655.

Tavits, Margit, and Natalia Letki. 2009. When left is right: Party ideology and policy in post-communist Europe. *American Political Science Review* 103 (4): 555–569.

Vukov, Visnja. 2016. The rise of the competition state? Transnationalization and state transformations in Europe. *Comparative European Politics* 14 (5): 523–546.

Weinerman, E. Richard. 1969. *Social medicine in Eastern Europe: The organization of health services and the education of medical personnel in Czechoslovakia, Hungary, and Poland*. Cambridge: Harvard University Press.

Weir, Margaret, and Theda Skocpol. 1985. State structures and the possibilities for 'Keynesian' responses to the great depression in Sweden, Britain and the United States. In *Bringing the state back in*, ed. Peter B. Evans, Dietrich Rueschemeyer, and Theda Skocpol. Cambridge: Cambridge University Press.

Williamson, John. 1990. What Washington means by policy reform. In *Latin American adjustment: How much has happened?* ed. J. Williamson, 5–20. Washington, DC: Institute for International Economics.

World Bank. 1990. *Poland: Health system reform: Meeting the challenge*. Washington, DC: World Bank.

———. 1991. *The Czech and Slovak federal republic: Issues and priorities in the healthcare sector*. Washington, DC: Europe and Central Asia, Middle East and North Africa Regions, Human Resource Operation Division.

Yee, Albert S. 1996. The causal effects of ideas on policies. *International Organizations* 50 (1): 69–108.

Ziblatt, Daniel F. 1998. The adaptation of ex-communist parties to post-communist East Central Europe: A comparative study of the East German and Hungarian ex-communist parties. *Communist and Post-Communist Studies* 31 (2): 119–137.

CHAPTER 3

Slovenia

Introduction

This chapter presents empirical evidence of the Slovenian health reforms over three post-communist decades. It accounts for the remarkably stable pattern of the country's healthcare policy path, explaining how market elements introduced in the country's health system during early transition managed to survive over time, despite challenges. The origins of the Slovenian market-oriented reforms, like those in Czech Republic and Poland, can be traced to the communist period. However, the Slovenian case is different because the idea of healthcare governed by market forces was already implemented under socialism through the introduction of a health system organisation based on workers' self-management. The resulting policy legacy included experience with the market-oriented provision of healthcare, and this was crucial for the post-communist reforms. Slovenian policymakers, similar to Czech and Polish reformers, embraced markets in health, but given their previous experiences with alternative modes of system organisation, they opted for a much more cautious and gradual approach to market reforms. The result of this approach is a healthcare system based on a state-market mix in which medical services are delivered almost exclusively through publicly owned healthcare facilities, but the financing of these services relies on a market instrument—complementary private insurance.

T. Popic, *Health Reforms in Post-Communist Eastern Europe*,
https://doi.org/10.1007/978-3-031-15497-3_3

The chapter shows how the remarkable persistence of this particular healthcare model throughout the transitional decades was enabled by the combination of an institutional setup featuring very few institutional veto points and weak conflict between political parties over health issues. This stability is puzzling, as the adopted policy model has been marked by controversy. For example, multiple attempts have been made to reform or eliminate complementary private insurance and the broader Slovenian public continues to question its fairness and equity (Hrast et al. 2018), yet all such attempts have failed.

From an institutional perspective, the Slovenian case is curious, a theoretical anomaly. The country's relatively light veto point structure may generate expectations of easy and frequent policy change, contributing to an unstable pattern (see Immergut 1990, 1992), but the healthcare policy has been quite stable. This underlines the importance of party conflict over healthcare—or in this case, its absence. In early transition, the lack of major party divisions over health policy issues was crucial for the establishment of the market-oriented policy model. Then, due to the path-dependent nature of policymaking within this specific political and institutional context, this model was left untouched in spite of attempts to abolish it and continuing public debate over its solidarity and fairness.

The chapter is organised as follows. It first accounts for policy developments of Slovenia's healthcare under socialism showing how after the successful post-war adaptation of the system to the Soviet health paradigm, policymakers experimented with market-oriented ideas under a specific model of healthcare organisation based on workers' self-management. It then offers an elaborate account of the post-communist reforms, focusing on four episodes: introduction of co-payments and complementary insurance, privatisation of primary care, and privatisation of hospitals. These reform episodes demonstrate how a combination of country-specific policy legacies, light institutional constraints and weak political party conflict over health issues shaped the gradual and successful incorporation of market ideas into the country's health system. The final section of the chapter provides a summary; it explains how Slovenia's policy experiences, politics and institutional factors shaped the process of policy learning that resulted in the country's unique healthcare policy path—the *survival* of a market-oriented healthcare model. As such, this experience stands in stark contrast to the Czech *instability* and Polish *reversal* of market reforms.

Slovenian Healthcare Under Socialism

Like other East European countries, Slovenia's health policy was strongly influenced by the Soviet healthcare paradigm during the early post-war period when the country became part of the Socialist Federal Republic of Yugoslavia (SFRY).[1] Healthcare provision was based on a hierarchical model, dominated by the state and grounded on the socialist principles of universalism and central planning, according to which medical care is to be delivered by the state through a strict vertical model of healthcare and provided universally. Even though the healthcare system closely adhered to the socialist paradigm, it had some unique features—it retained the insurance system established during the inter-war period and a strong focus on primary care. With the transformation of Yugoslav socialism in the 1950s and the 1960s, a new model emerged. Based on workers' self-management, the model stressed strong decentralisation, a large degree of institutional autonomy and responsiveness to patients' needs as core principles of healthcare management. Yet, as the anomalies of this new self-managed system became evident, a policy crisis ensued, instigating discussions on the appropriate role of state and market in healthcare provision, and these, in turn, built the basis for the ensuing post-communist reform debate.

Introduction of the Socialist Policy Paradigm

Following World War II, Slovenia became part of socialist federal Yugoslavia. The Communist Party of Slovenia, an autonomous sub-branch of the Yugoslav communist party, the League of Communists of Yugoslavia, was the only legal party in the country. As a member of the federation, Slovenia shared a healthcare policy with the five other Yugoslav republics. The main focus of the early post-war health policy in SFRY was the establishment of a universal, state-dominated and centralised system of healthcare provision (Albreht et al. 2002, 2009). The first important post-war health law, the 1945 Law on Implementation of Social Insurance, integrated existing social insurance institutions throughout SFRY and centralised healthcare financing (Popic 2021). It established the Central Institute for Social Insurance, an institution with insurance branches at the level of

[1] Slovenia was part of SFRY from 1945 to 1991.

the republics; in Slovenia, this was the Federal Institute for Social Insurance (*Federalni zavod za socialno zavarovanje—FZSZ*).

Centralisation of healthcare financing was one of the core principles of SFRY's post-war health policy; even though the country was formally a federation, the central administration dominated the healthcare financing of the republics. The post-war system initially privileged the industrial working class, but gradually extended healthcare coverage to the rest of the population, thus fulfilling the socialist principle of universality. A series of federal laws introduced throughout the late 1940s and the 1950s extended coverage to other occupational groups, public employees and officials, as well as agricultural workers (Popic and Perišić 2021).[2]

Another series of laws at the level of the Slovenian republic introduced changes in healthcare delivery, similarly inspired by the state-dominated model.[3] Centralisation implied nationalisation through transfer of the property rights of healthcare institutions to the central state (Parmelee et al. 1982; Parmelee 1985). Private practice of medicine was suspended in 1947 and banned completely in 1957 (Albreht and Klazinga 2009),[4] a policy move coupled with the abolition of the Slovenian Medical Chamber. As a consequence, healthcare institutions became the property of the state, and healthcare professionals were now salaried state employees. Those professionals who resisted transition from private to public services were threatened with sanctions (Dobaja 2009). Once employed as civil servants, doctors and other healthcare workers were assigned to a state health facility, and their professional autonomy became severely restricted (Albreht et al. 2002, 2009; Albreht 2011).

The post-war changes of the Slovenian health policy hence implied a close modelling of the Soviet socialist policy paradigm (see also Estrin 1991). According to the communist party leadership, the shift to centralised, state-governed healthcare services was part of the battle for the liquidation of private and capitalist elements in the health sector to pave the

[2] 1946 Law on Social Insurance of Workers, Public Employees, and Officials; 1950 Law on Social Insurance of Workers and Employees and their Families; 1959 Law on Health Insurance for Agricultural Workers (Popic and Perišić 2021: 906).

[3] 1956 Law on Medical Centres and Medical Stations (*Zakon o zdravstvenih domovi in zdravstvenih postajah*); 1956 Law on Hospitals (*Zakon o bolnicah*).

[4] 1957 Law on Private Health Practice in the People's Republic of Slovenia (*Zakon o zasebni zdravstveni praksi v Ljudski Republiki Sloveniji*). After 1957, private practice continued to a limited extent as a 'grey market' activity, predominantly amongst dentists (Albreht and Klazinga 2009).

way for the establishment of 'State Socialist relations' (Dobaja 2009). Within this broader socialist paradigm, state-dominated, centrally organised, and publicly delivered medical care was seen as the most effective model of healthcare organisation and superior to market alternatives.

Yet, Slovenia's healthcare model was unique in the Eastern Bloc. Following World War II, most countries in the region simply transplanted the Soviet 'Semashko' system of healthcare. Slovenia's model differed from the Soviet one in two respects. First, despite the shift to the state-dominated and centrally organised system, the country preserved its insurance system of healthcare financing established during the inter-war period. This meant the health system was not financed through the state budget, as in the Semashko system, but through the insurance contributions of both employers and employees (Albreht et al. 2002).

Second, the Slovenian healthcare model focused on primary care, based on the 'Štampar model' (Brown and Fee 2006).[5] This model dated back to the 1920s and emphasised social medicine, which meant strengthening public health, including both primary and preventive care (Himmelstein et al. 1984). Its organisation was based on a network of public community health centres (*zdravstveni domovi*) which delivered a broad range of primary care services, including general practice, paediatrics, medicine for school children and adolescents, occupational medicine, pulmonary care, gynaecology, dentistry, and physical therapy. The focus on primary care was particularly strong in Slovenia, compared to the other Yugoslav republics (Albreht et al. 2002, 2009). The country also took the lead in the development of a healthcare workforce and infrastructure, as it featured a relatively high number of doctors and hospital beds compared to the other republics. These developments were linked to impressive achievements in population health outcomes, with indicators such as infant mortality showing dramatic improvement by the 1960s (Parmelee 1989).

The different nature of the Slovenian post-war health system had a political basis as well. Yugoslavia was the only Eastern Bloc country to break with Soviet style policies very early, with a split opening up between the country's leader Josip Broz Tito and Soviet leader Joseph Stalin in 1948 (Parmelee et al. 1982). Following this split, there was no pressure to closely adhere to the Soviet model, and policymakers were able to retain

[5] 'Štampar model' was named after Dr. Andrija Štampar, the head of the Department of Public Health in the Kingdom of Yugoslavia, a strong advocate of social medicine (Brown and Fee 2006).

some of the country's pre-war institutional arrangements, such as the insurance model of healthcare financing and the focus on primary care. This particular political context was responsible for the unique features of the country's health system and allowed greater flexibility to depart from the more common, centralised, state-run health systems of the early post-war period.

Emergence of Market Idea: Shift to Workers' Self-Management

Despite significant achievements in coverage, healthcare infrastructure and population health outcomes, the socialist state-centred healthcare system generated an inflexible model of healthcare organisation. The provision of medical care was hierarchical, as the system was managed by the central state which distributed healthcare resources following a five-year plan rather than according to actual population needs (Field 1989). This model of healthcare management reflected the overall socio-economic model of the socialist state based on strict vertical command planning and centralised distribution of resources (Estrin 1991).

The first steps towards changing the post-war policy model were taken in the 1950s. The 1953 Constitutional Law loosened certain federal regulations and introduced the core principles of a new model of socio-economic organisation—workers' self-management.[6] The origins of the self-managed model dated back to 1948, when Tito split politically from the Soviet leadership, and this, in turn, led to Yugoslavia's decisive break from the influence of the Soviet Union. Tito shifted from a 'hard' state-centred socialism to a 'soft' socialism which included experimentation with an autonomous socio-economic model of socialism—workers' self-management (Parmelee et al. 1982; Himmelstein et al. 1984). The move towards 'soft' socialism took place with the 1963 Constitution,[7] which re-designed Yugoslavia as a federal state. Under this Constitution, the republics were given a significant degree of autonomy in socio-economic matters, including healthcare. The 1974 Constitution took a major move towards an even looser federation, as it delegated control over most public sectors, including healthcare, to the republics. Medical services were no longer defined at the federal level,

[6] 1953 Constitutional law on the basis of the social and political structure of SFRY.

[7] 1963 Constitution of SFRY.

and workers' self-management was designated the main principle of socio-economic organisation (Albreht 2011).[8]

The core principles of the self-managed model were decentralisation and autonomy. The underlying idea was that citizens should be able to define their needs and determine the ways in which these needs should be satisfied without the intervention of the central state (Markota and Albreht 2001). In healthcare, self-management meant medical care was financed through a complex model of non-governmental, locally responsible, administrative institutions—'self-managing communities of interest' (*samoupravne interesne skupnosti—SIS*). These communities were organised around a well-defined territory and had two councils of elected delegates—one representing local healthcare providers and the other representing local healthcare users. In practice, this meant local associations in communities with a population of at least 150,000 handled all issues related to the financing of healthcare insurance in their area (Šarić and Rodwin 1993).

In healthcare delivery, departure from the centralised system led to the establishment of regional community health centres. These were expected to provide a full range of preventive and curative services and thus included hospitals, primary health centres, pharmacies, and the respective regional institutes of public health (Albreht et al. 2002).

Within healthcare facilities, workers' self-management became the main model of management and organisation. Healthcare workers were no longer state employees, and instead of being assigned to a specific facility, they were free to seek positions as they became available and advertised. Health facilities became autonomous from the state and were self-managed by their employees and community representatives (Parmelee et al. 1982). In practice, this meant a healthcare facility, for example, a hospital, was administered through a management council; two-thirds of council member were employees and one-third external members. The main task of these councils was to plan healthcare delivery based on local needs, setting fee schedules, opening and closing services and adding new healthcare personnel (Berg et al. 1976; Kunitz 1979). In addition, all health institutions had worker assemblies which included all those working in the institution. These assemblies were responsible for the final approval of the budget and were involved in the selection of an institution's directors. The

[8] 1974 Constitution of SFRY and the constitutions of the socialist republics and autonomous provinces.

principle of autonomy was also evident, in that the specific departments within a healthcare institution were able to make up their own budgets and present them to the director; in addition, the healthcare workers within each department could establish their own salaries (Kunitz 1979).

The Socialist Healthcare Crisis

Workers' self-management has been considered a distinctive feature of Yugoslav socialism. It was softer than the Soviet paradigm of central planning and the state-dominated model of social and economic organisation (Estrin 1991). In the self-managed model, healthcare was expected to function on the basis of the core principle of autonomy but was also expected to be efficient. Healthcare facilities were seen as similar to productive enterprises in other sectors of the economy operating on the principle of net income, as the model emphasised the importance of efficient management of existing resources (Kunitz 1979). The introduction of self-management in healthcare was also seen as tool to improve the accessibility of health services, as its focus on local needs was supposed to allow a closer fit between these needs and service delivery, along with greater participation of users and providers in healthcare decision-making (Parmelee et al. 1982).

By the late 1970s, however, it was clear that rather than solving the problems of the socialist state, the self-managed model generated new ones. In healthcare, a general issue was how the model worked in practice. As a theoretical concept, self-management was appealing, but there were discrepancies between the idealised concept of workers' self-management in healthcare service production and the realities of daily management practice. The introduction of self-management in the provision of medical services implied a vast increase in bureaucracy, as non-medical professionals gradually took over the management of the system (Markota and Albreht 2001). Healthcare facilities were increasingly dominated by technically trained experts and thus were decreasingly responsive to community control. This ran counter to the theoretical focus on local needs (Kunitz 1979).

Another problem was that rather than being efficient, the focus on self-management resulted in a highly fragmented and dysfunctional model of healthcare organisation. With decentralisation, local facilities pursued their own self-interests, and this meant a lack of functional links between facilities. Even within the same facility, for example, child dispensaries and children's hospital departments could function as separate institutions (Kunitz 1979). Healthcare activities developed in many small independent units without knowledge of or concern about what was going on in other units, making any type of planning of service provision impossible. As each community of interests had its own policy that was appropriate for the local level but not for the systemic level, the result was fragmentation and duplication of services, technology and staff, generating inequalities in the scope and quality of care and suboptimal use of available resources (Himmelstein et al. 1984).

In theory, self-management implied healthcare institutions were fully autonomous *vis-à-vis* the state, but the reality was different. Officially, healthcare workers were authorised to select members for the workers' council and management board from their ranks. The workers' councils, unlike other sectors of the economy, also included representatives of the local government and local political bodies. This model was never fully implemented, however, as most health institutions were established directly by the municipal or the national government; thus, the state still played a very important role in the process of resource allocation. The local government influenced the decision-making process in health facilities through the government representatives on the workers' councils. No decision on capital expenditures could be made without the approval of the majority of external members of the council. As a result, healthcare workers were autonomous only in managing day-to-day activities.

The autonomy of the self-managing communities of interests was similarly restricted by the state. Representatives of healthcare providers and users agreed on the insurance contributions from employers and employees; these were then established by the administrative unit of the community of interest, approved by local government and rubber-stamped by the councils. However, the maximum annual rate of contributions was regulated by the national and federal governments. Hence, despite the goal to increase the participation of local communities and users of healthcare services, their influence on the decision-making process was minimal (Parmelee 1985; Šarić and Rodwin 1993).

Moreover, in theory, the autonomy of health facilities implied they could hire and fire workers without the permission of the state, and healthcare professionals would be paid according to a pay-scale developed by each facility. In reality, however, national and federal laws required facilities to hire new workers irrespective of the need for new staff in order to reduce unemployment rates amongst healthcare professionals. Other legal regulations made firing of healthcare staff impossible, and the federal government was able to freeze salaries, whilst the national government regulated the range between the highest and lowest salary within a facility.[9] In sum, state intervention in a self-managed model was the rule rather than the exception, with healthcare institutions ending up as powerless appendages to the government (Šarić and Rodwin 1993; see also Berg et al. 1976; Kunitz 1979).

The self-managed healthcare model demonstrated the risks of both market and state failures; leaving healthcare provision to local forces engendered risks, but state control exposed the standard weaknesses of the socialist planned economy. As a result of multiple failures, by the late 1970s, some serious anomalies of the self-managed healthcare model became apparent.

As the socialist economy declined, health systems faced problems all across the Soviet Bloc (Parmelee 1985). Healthcare financing gradually decreased; in Slovenia, the percentage of the social product spent on healthcare dropped from 5.7 to 4.7 per cent from 1979 to 1986 (Komadina 1988). In this fragmented yet universal system, patients had almost unlimited rights to an unlimited set of services; not surprisingly, the system became financially unsustainable. Whilst citizens were entitled to almost any type of service, the health system saw increasing tension between progressively more expensive health service on the one hand and the low system funding and efficiency on the other. With rapidly growing signs of economic, managerial and social crisis, by the 1980s, the Slovenian health system was on the verge of collapse (Markota and Albreht 2001; Albreht 2011).

The first reaction to the crisis was to shift healthcare financing onto patients. In 1978, the socialist government introduced patient co-payments, arguing they would raise patients' awareness of the actual costs of care, increase responsibility and prevent patients from seeking unnecessary care.[10] The co-payments, in popular parlance called 'participations', required patients to 'participate' in financing part of the costs of delivered

[9] By law, the salary of the highest paid worker could not be more than five times the salary of the lowest paid worker within an institution (Berg et al. 1976).

[10] The co-payments were introduced in the 1980 Law on Healthcare (*Zakon o zdravstvenem varstvu, Uradni list SRS, 1/80*) and further defined and regulated in amendment in 1982 and 1984 (*Zakon o spremembah in dopolnitvah zakona o zdravstvenem varstvu, Uradni list SRS, 45/82*; *Zakon o spremembah in dopolnitvah zakona o zdravstvenem varstvu, Uradni list SRS, 45/84*).

services The list of services requiring co-payments initially included only specific services but was gradually expanded; by the end of the 1980s, it included a wide range of services, covering even regular visits to doctors and some forms of acute hospital care, with exemptions for specific categories such as war veterans and patients with chronic diseases (Jošt-Doma 1983; see also Šarić and Rodwin 1993).

These policy changes did not halt the criticism of the existing healthcare model. Although they admitted there were 'theoretical' advantages of the state's role in the healthcare sector, critics emphasised that the existing system, despite its market-oriented elements, showed all the weaknesses of state monopoly (see Boh 1989). One of the major weaknesses, in their view, was an overly bureaucratic health system with an oversized management apparatus that ran counter to the original idea of the self-managed model as able to reduce the role of the state. One critic commented:

> The first weakness is the bureaucratized management apparatus. … Expectations that the introduction of SIS's [self-managed communities of interests] … will reduce the influence of the state and foster users' participation in the decision-making process did not materialize. Instead of reducing the impact of management to simplify decision-making, reducing costs and increasing influence of users, the developments went in the opposite direction. We got an oversized control apparatus … which is blocked, left without feedback, inefficient and not adapted to real needs. (Boh 1989: 3)[11]

Interestingly, these views were contrary to external advice. Foreign experts who visited Yugoslavia in the 1980s blamed decentralisation of healthcare financing for the problems of the health sector, arguing the extensive degree of local autonomy inherent to self-management was the main source of problems. As a remedy, they suggested returning state control through the re-introduction of 'central state coordination' (Parmelee 1985). This suggestion was bluntly rejected by the country's policy experts who argued that whilst the state may have a constructive role in the development of a healthcare system, it also has limits, as demonstrated by the country's own socialist experience (Milanović and Stambolović 1985).

[11] The author of this critical review was Katja Boh, who became the head of the parliamentary Committee for Health and Social Welfare in the first Slovenian democratic government formed in 1990 and was the Minister of Heath from 1990 to 1991 in Peterle's government.

The Slovenian healthcare policy debate intensified in the second half of the 1980s. Continued critical appraisals of the system showed deep disillusionment with socialism, even in its self-managed form. Some claimed the crisis had destroyed the illusion that socialism could afford to provide healthcare equally to all on the basis of solidarity (Svetlik 1989). They suggested the functioning of the healthcare system could be improved through an appropriate combination of the state and the market's commercial sector. This would imply replacement of the 'quasi-state monopoly' with a more pluralistic model, including not only public, but also commercial, corporatist and informal sectors. In particular, the shift to the commercial sector was seen as predicting the abolition of the state monopoly and higher efficiency, as well as increased patient choice. Together, these would result in more freedom and equality (Svetlik 1989; see also Boh 1989; Cernić Istenić 1998).

The experts' views on policy reforms were nuanced. They pointed out advantages and potential problems in the different approaches. The advantage of the public sector was that it could guarantee patients' right of access and procedural rights related to the use of medical services, but as its dominance could generate inefficiencies, they suggested the state should play a regulatory role. The experts stressed policymakers should be aware of other types of monopolies and their dangers; for example, a monopoly of doctors could easily increase demand for health services (Svetlik 1989). They also warned about problems caused by asymmetries of information and possible inequalities generated through market allocation:

> For example, due to mutual competition, all hospitals want to be equipped with the latest equipment, which is not fully used. The users of services often do not have the necessary information to really be able to choose between different services and make rational decisions. For these reasons, the question arises as to what place the market should play in the provision of services. Is it necessary to strive to expand the market allocation of services, or should we try to eliminate as many market imperfections as possible, or should we try to take into account market principles as much as possible when it comes to state programs. (Svetlik 1989: 7)[12]

[12] The author of this critical review was Ivan Svetlik, future Minister of Labour, Family and Social Affairs in Slovenia's post-communist government under Borut Pahor (2008–2011).

Overall, the critical consensus was that a future healthcare system should be a combination of public and private elements (Cernić Istenić 1998). Advocates for change stressed the need for a balanced and coordinated approach in policy reforms, arguing the main issue was not the sector, but how to use the advantages of each sector and combine their elements, whilst taking into consideration their interactions and synergetic effects (Svetlik 1989; see also Cernić Istenić 1998).

Institutional and Political Context of Post-Communist Health Reform

Slovenian policy debate under socialism demonstrated a high degree of awareness of state and, even more importantly, market failures in the healthcare sector. Policymakers had experience with both 'hard' Soviet socialism and the 'soft' version of socialism embodied in a market-like, self-managed model. Thus, in contrast to their Czech and Polish colleagues, during post-communism, they took a deliberate but more cautious approach to market reforms. From a policy point of view, this implied a relatively smooth learning process through which market ideas could be integrated into the provision of medical services, generating institutional lock-ins and path-dependent policy development (Popic 2021).

The comparatively smoother departure of Slovenian healthcare from a state to a market-oriented model and its stability were due to the country's post-communist context. The contextual factors underpinning the policy stability were twofold: the institutional architecture of the new Slovenian state and the nature of the political party competition emerging during the country's transition to democracy. With respect to the former, SFRY was dissolved, and the 1991 Constitution of Slovenian as now an independent state established institutional configurations with few vetoes and strong corporatist elements. With respect to the latter, the early post-communist policymaking was marked by cross-party consensus on core policy issues, resulting in weak political conflict over healthcare reforms. This also enabled parties to dominate the various healthcare interests and selectively use these interests in the context of social dialogue (see also Fink-Hafner 1998). The main result of these institutional and political arrangements was a resilient pattern of healthcare policy development characterised by the absence of reform reversals despite multiple attempts to eliminate market elements from the system.

Institutions: Light Veto Points Configurations

The 1991 Constitution delineated the institutional setup of the new Slovenian state. It established a bicameral parliament consisting of the Lower House, the National Assembly (*Državni Zbor*), and the Upper House, the National Council (*Državni Svet*), in an 'asymmetric' institutional structure (see Guardiancich 2012). The Assembly was composed of members of the political parties, and the Council was composed of members of local entities and social categories, including representatives of local interests and social, economic, trade and professional groups (Constitution of the Republic of Slovenia 1991, Art. 96).[13]

This parliamentary structure was also asymmetric in its veto arrangements. The Lower House was given the right to prepare and pass bills with a majority of votes, whilst the Upper House received significantly weaker and conditional veto power. Its veto of bills passed in the Lower House was defined a conditional on the support of the absolute majority of the House's votes (Constitution of the Republic of Slovenia 1991, Art. 97). In addition, the nature of the Upper House's veto was rigidly defined; it had to reject a law in its entirety, not partially, even if it opposed only one part of the law. The Upper House was also given an extremely short period to examine the laws passed by the Lower House—seven days (Constitution of the Republic of Slovenia 1991, Art. 91).[14] Given these limits on the veto powers of the Upper House, Slovenian bicameralism has been defined as 'masked' (Fasone 2019) or simply 'weak' (Štrus 2019; see also Passaglia 2018).[15]

The decision-making powers of the Lower House were not significantly curtailed by the powers of the President of the Republic either, as the President was given no power to veto bills passed by Parliament. The 1991 Constitution gave additional veto competencies only to the electorate and

[13] The National Council consists of 22 representatives of local interests and 18 representatives of socio-economic groups: 4 representatives of employers, 4 representatives of employees, 4 representatives of farmers, crafts and trades, and independent professions, and 6 representatives of non-commercial fields (Constitution of the Republic of Slovenia 1991, Art. 96).

[14] In contrast, Czech Republic's and Poland's upper houses have 30 days to examine the law (Constitution of the Republic of Poland, Art. 121; Constitution of the Czech Republic of 16 December 1992, Art. 46.).

[15] The powers of the Council versus the powers of the Assembly are deeply disputed. The dispute has led to a reduction of some of the Council's powers; for example, the 2013 constitutional amendment eliminated the right of the Council to call for a legislative referendum (Štrus 2019).

the Constitutional Court, who were allowed to veto laws through a public referendum and a constitutional review, respectively (Constitution of the Republic of Slovenia 1991, Art. 90 and Art. 156). The consequence of this specific institutional structure was that healthcare policymaking developed primarily within the government and the Lower House (see also Fink-Hafner and Krašovec 2005), with the only possible checks on its decisions coming from the Court or the electorate.

Another important element of the new institutional architecture was corporatism. The post-communist period saw a rebirth of the socialist corporatist tradition, with the institutional setup formally assigning a specifically defined space for interest groups to influence the policymaking process (Fink-Hafner 1998). The composition of the National Council was one of the main corporatist elements of the new system, but another formally established channel of interest group influence on policymaking was the Economic and Social Council (*Ekonomski in socialni svet*). Its strongly neo-corporatist structure consisted of three delegations representing the three partners: labour, business, and the state. As such, it was meant to foster tripartism and social dialogue, with its views on economic and social policies formally channelled to the government, the parliament and the public. The corporatist influence in policymaking was formalised in the role of professional chambers, which were given specific competencies in the creation and implementation of public policies through the activities of the parliamentary working bodies.

Because of these multiple formal channels of interest group influence on policymaking, the Slovenian policymaking context has been called neo-corporatist (Lukšić 2003; Fink-Hafner 1998, 2019; Fink-Hafner and Krašovec 2005; Guardiancich 2012; Krašovec and Johannsen 2016). Yet, even with an elaborate neo-corporatist structure in place, the influence of corporatist interests on health policy was selective and mediated by political parties (see also Fink-Hafner 1998). Representatives of employers' organisations, trade unions, insurance companies, healthcare professionals and other interest groups were regularly invited to participate in meetings and parliamentary working sessions on health reforms, but the parties in the government were only selectively open to social dialogue and consultative politics in the policymaking process. For example, in the context of health insurance reforms, the government resisted changes to the existing market-oriented model reliant on the complementary private insurance (2003, 2011), thus supporting insurance companies' interests. Yet, the government also decided to limit the companies' autonomy in the use of profit and setting of insurance premiums (2005). This illustrates 'selective corporatism' in which government acted as a gate-keeper and depending on its own policy preferences could selectively strengthen or weaken the voice of interest groups in the policymaking process (see Fink-Hafner 1998; see also Fink-Hafner and Krašovec 2005).

Party Politics: Weak Party Divide on Health Policy

The building of the post-communist political system began with the 1989 amendments to the Constitution. These provided the basis for a multi-party system and democratic elections. The country's political transformation took place in the framework of a new independent state, grounded on the December 1990 referendum, followed by an official proclamation of the country's independence from SFRY on 25 June 1991. The passing of the constitutional amendment, the preparation of the referendum and rather elegant separation from SFRY were seen as a result of close cooperation between the old communist reformers and the emerging opposition (Zajc 2013).

The development of the Slovenian party system was marked by relative stability. The main cleavage defining the post-communist party arena and its structure especially during the first transitional decades was the communism–anticommunism cleavage (O'Dwyer 2014). The important issue was the question of existence during the socialist period; parties were differentiated as (post-)communist or 'new' parties, the latter being the opposition parties established in the 1980s during the period of liberalisation. The result was competition between the cluster of 'old' centre-left parties and the cluster of 'new' predominately centre-right parties (Cabada 2005; Fink-Hafner 2006).

The 'old' cluster was dominated by a centre-left party with liberal leanings, the Liberal Democratic Party (LDS).[16] The LDS originated in the former Federation of the Socialist Youth of Slovenia (*Zveza socialistične mladine Slovenije, ZSMS*), an independent organisation with liberal values, such as individual rights and freedoms (Bugajski 2002). During the 1980s, the Federation become a voice for civil society demanding democratic changes; in the post-communist context, the LDS was seen as the successor

[16] In 1994, the party changed its name to Liberal Democracy of Slovenia, retaining its acronym (LDS).

to the 'systemic opposition' under the old regime. This understanding enabled party leader Janez Drnovšek to shift LDS's identity from a communist into a left-oriented liberal party (Fink-Hafner 2006). Successfully transforming in the new political context, the LDS enjoyed broad popular support. It became the dominant party on the country's political landscape during the first decade and a half of the post-communist period.

Thanks to its pivotal position within the party system, the LDS facilitated a relatively smooth transition from socialism to capitalism and private ownership and was largely successful in implementing its social and economic programme. It pursued moderately liberal policies in both social and economic terms and was seen as occupying the middle of the political spectrum. This enabled it to moderate the conflict between the left and right and to form a number of 'mixed' government coalitions (Krašovec and Haughton 2011; Zajc 2013).

Another important 'old' party on the left side of the political spectrum was the United List of Social Democrats (ZLSD/SD).[17] In contrast to the left-liberal LDS, the ZLSD was technically a communist successor party as it was formed by a coalition of several groups derived from the former ruling League of Communists (*Zveza komunistov Slovenije, ZKS*) and its various fronts (Zajc 2013). The ZLSD initially focused on protecting the 'gains of socialism', but knowing its survival depended on adaptation to the new political context, it took a new approach to these gains and strongly criticised the communist regime. Over time, it added neo-corporatism and the welfare state to the list of the party goals, along with a set of modern and post-modern values, including environmental and gender equality. As a result, the party managed to make a clean break with its communist past, casting its identity as equivalent to that of Tony Blair's New Labour and marketing itself as a party of the middle rather than a party of the left. Adopting the 'Third Way' identity allowed it to differentiate itself from both the liberals and the right-wing parties—a wise move, as it turned out to be a successful electoral strategy (Zajc 2013; Cabada 2005).

On the right, the most electorally successful party was a 'new' party called the Social Democratic Party (SDSS/SDS).[18] Interestingly, the SDS started out as a party of the left and ended up as a party of the right. It was

[17] In 2005, the party changed its name to Social Democrats (*Socialni Demokrati—SD*).

[18] In 2003, the party changed its name to Slovenian Democratic Party (*Slovenska demokratska stranka—SDS*).

created in the late 1980s as one of the 'Slovenian spring' parties pushing for democratic reform and subsequently independence; in the post-communist period, it initially described itself as a social democratic party in the tradition of European democracy and the social state. Despite its social democratic label, favouring fast-paced market reforms and speaking out against ex-communists, the party quickly shifted to the right (Bugajski 2002). Over time, the SDS became one of the major political players on the right, drawing more than 25 per cent of electoral votes (Zajc 2013) and emerging as the main competitor of the LDS. However, its success was overshadowed by scandals.[19]

Despite the ideological differences, the Slovenian party dynamic during early transition was marked by inter-party cooperation across ideological lines (Fink-Hafner 2006). A very important factor was the parties' common focus on the changing environment. Through institutionalisation and gradual maturation, both the 'old' and the 'new' parties were expected to adapt to the environment by becoming less ideologically focused on the on-going change and more concentrated on developing a pragmatic approach to building broader electoral support (Fink-Hafner 2006: 216). As a consequence, the parties developed a tendency to move towards the centre, so that in spite of the communist versus anti-communist cleavage, fairly stable, ideologically mixed, grand coalition governments were formed.[20] In addition to government coalitions, the parties also often formed parliamentary coalitions; this was part of the strategy of LDS leader Drnovšek, who used his party's political dominance to overcome ideological polarisations. This strategy was successful; despite the ideologically mixed coalitions, Slovenian governments were seen as amongst the most stable in the region, and the country's transition was qualified as marked by consensualism, pragmatism, and gradualism (Lindstrom and Piroška 2004; see also O'Dwyer 2014; Krašovec and Johannsen 2016).[21]

This general pattern was destabilised in 2004, when the LDS lost to the SDS and subsequently plunged into decline and fragmentation. On the left, the LDS was replaced first by the ZLSD/SD and then by new parties,

[19] In 2014, SDS leader Janez Janša spent six months in prison after being convicted on bribery charges related to a 2006 arms deal.

[20] Six out of nine governments during 1990–2010 were grand coalitions (Guardiancich 2012).

[21] Slovenia enjoyed the highest per capita GDP in the whole post-communist bloc; this has been singled out as a reason why the market–redistributive policy differences were not the primary markers in the field of party competition (O'Dwyer 2014).

the Positive Slovenia (*Pozitivna Slovenia—PS*), and the Modern Centre Party (*Stranka Modernega Centra—SMC*). As the right become dominated by the SDS, led by Janez Janša, amicable cooperation turned into bipolarity and fragmentation; centre-left and centre-right clusters of parties had problems creating ideologically coherent government coalitions. The political climate had changed; polarisation grew with the increasing electoral success of the SDS. As a result, rather than governing with majorities from both sides of political spectrum, governing was based on small majorities from either the right or the left side of the spectrum, and grand coalitions became a thing of the past (Krašovec and Johannsen 2016; Guardiancich 2012). This political pattern remained unchanged in the 2008 global economic crisis, with other episodes of party system destabilisation, such as the one in 2011, resulting in early elections, a pattern repeated in 2014 and 2018.

Nevertheless, the main effect of the Slovenian post-communist politics on health policy development over the three transitional decades was stability characterised by an absence of systemic reforms. The three parties dominating the political landscape during the initial transition—the LDS, the ZLSD, and the SD—all had socialist origins, albeit different, and in an effort to build their new post-communist identity, they were prone to espousing moderately liberal transition programmes (Krašovec and Haughton 2011). Taking a gradualist approach and aware of the population's clear expectation of retaining the welfare state, all parliamentary parties advocated similar socio-economic policies (Stanojević and Krašovec 2011). Consequently, particularly during the early transition, the intensity of party dissention on health issues was low. The party dominating Slovenian politics during the formative health reforms in early transition, the LDS, was an 'old' communist party but was now pragmatically focused on successful adaptation to the new political context. The changes to the health system put forward by the LDS in the early 1990s featured a combination of private insurance as a market element in financing and a system of health services still provided by the state; these moderately liberal policy options allowed consensual policymaking even in ideologically mixed coalitions.

In the second and third post-communist decades, increased political polarisation and party fragmentation were evident in the attempts to abolish the complementary private insurance. Yet, the lack of real inter-party conflict over health—of the type evidenced in the case of Polish and, to a lesser extent, Czech health reforms—was reflected in the fact that proposals for the abolition of private insurance came from intra-party ranks of the LDS, and as these proposals lacked broader political backing, the healthcare policy model remained unchanged. Even with the increased political fragmentation and instability in the wake of the 2008 financial crisis, private insurance and public delivery were generally seen as key elements of healthcare system stability.[22] Hence, even though Slovenia was strongly affected by the crisis, there was no major division over health issues and, hence, no major reforms.

The existence of a consensual model of policymaking in early transition was key to stable policy development, and it allowed a smooth process of policy learning. The initial political consensus on health policy meant the government's reform decisions were not politically contested, and new elements could easily be adopted. The consensus also enabled selective corporatism, whereby political parties acted as gatekeepers of corporatist interests, allowing interest groups such as private insurance companies some concessions but not others and consistently preventing doctors from influencing the reform process in healthcare delivery. The combination of these country-specific political and institutional dynamics contributed to a path-dependent policy development and institutional lock-ins. This, in turn, allowed the gradual adaptation of a market-oriented policy model and promoted its survival over time.

Key Episodes in Post-Communist Healthcare Reform

Initial Post-Communist Healthcare Reform Debates

Slovenia's first free multiparty parliamentary elections took place in April 1990 and resulted in the defeat of the former Communist party and the victory of the Democratic Opposition of Slovenia (DEMOS), a coalition of five anti-communist political parties.[23] The DEMOS coalition won almost 55 per cent of votes for Socio-political Chamber, with the United List of Social Democrats (ZLSD) emerging as the largest party, winning 14 of the Chamber's seats. Subsequently, the coalition formed a government under Lojze Peterle as Prime Minister. DEMOS' victory marked the beginning of the post-communist period and opened the door to debate

[22] Interview No.1.

[23] These first elections took place within the federal and institutional framework of the SFRJ.

on the future of the country's health system. Breakup with the past was signalled by the appointment of Katja Boh, one of the vocal critics of the socialist health system in the 1980s, as the Minister of Health, Family and Social Welfare in Peterle's government. This appointment also signalled the continuity of ideas, as it built on discussions initiated in late socialism—notably those expressing disillusionment with the socialist model of healthcare and requesting viable market alternatives.

Amongst the critics of the self-managed model was Minister of Legislation Lojze Janko. He argued the socialist model was built on the erroneous assumption that a system based on communities of interests without the state as an intermediary would ensure efficient performance and coordination between individual and general social interests (Janko 1990). Instead of coordination, Janko said, the result was a system that was fragmented, extremely complex, cumbersome and lacking control. Another consequence of self-management was the state's withdrawal from the provision of public services; these responsibilities were transferred to self-managed communities of interests, but they could not cope with the given tasks. The withdrawal of the state also resulted in concepts such as public finances, public funding and public administration being forgotten. The Minister warned that the new system would have to correct for these deficiencies, whilst simultaneously adopting market elements. In healthcare, this implied a return to a more standardised insurance model that would rely on both compulsory and voluntary health insurance schemes, clearly defining the role of the private sector (Janko 1990).

Janko's views reflected a general agreement with the architecture of a new health system organised according to the insurance model with private elements,[24] but also pointed to problematic aspects of the public–private model of healthcare provision. The major concerns were the specific forms of health insurance, the related issue of public–private sharing in the coverage of healthcare costs, the position of private health practitioners and the state's regulating role (Cernić Istenić 1998). Another concern was privatisation of primary care. Božidar Voljč, the head of the parliamentary Health Committee (and later Minister of Health), considered this a sensitive issue, as shifting primary care from public to private hands ran the risk of ruining the relatively well-functioning networks of public community health centres (Voljč 1991).[25] Taken together, these concerns showed

[24] Interview No. 3.
[25] Interview No. 2.

critical awareness of both the deficiencies and the qualities of the socialist system, as they criticised the self-managed model but were careful not to 'throw out the baby with the bath water' (see Barr 1994: 290).

Yet, the architects of reform also argued one of the guiding principles of health reform should be market-like incentives, based on the idea that money in health should 'finally get its true value' (Voljč 1991). This meant adequate pay of health professionals by insurance companies and patients' involvement in healthcare costs through co-payments. The latter could also be used to regulate demand for medical services (Voljč 1991). At the same time, the critics warned the reformers of the broader social and economic implications of the market-oriented system and the risks of the healthcare system turning into a profit-making sector, pointing out:

> We must take into account that healthcare in principle can be organized as a commodity-market relationship, because the buyer is a consumer of health services, the seller is a provider of health services and the subject of exchange are health services. However, the fact that provision of health services is only one general condition of modern production should not be overlooked. The effect of health services is not only a subjective increase in well-being, but also contribution to the economic development of society (…) As a result, it is not possible to leave the healthcare activities to the uncontrollable commodity market, which aims primarily at maximizing profits and not at meeting collective needs. (Brus 1990: 301)

As these comments suggest, the debate on the architecture of the new system was strongly influenced by previous experience with the market-like elements within the self-managed model. Policymakers were able to critically evaluate the use of markets in healthcare provision and thus advocated a balanced approach. This meant keeping the good elements of the old system and not privatising healthcare delivery based on community health centres. At the same time, changes in healthcare financing should involve a shift to an insurance system that would be recentralised and gradually combined with market elements—first, a wide range of patient co-payments for health services and then, complementary private health insurance (see also Cernić Istenić 1998).

Introduction of Social Health Insurance and Co-payments for Health Services

Peterle's government, composed of the DEMOS coalition, and with Božidar Voljč as the Minister of Health, was responsible for initiating the gradual shift to a new system. The first healthcare reform was introduced in the 1992 Law on Healthcare and Health Insurance. [26] This law shifted the existing insurance model into a more standard system with a Bismarckian insurance base, stipulating health insurance would be administered by the Health Insurance Institute of Slovenia (HIIS), a public and not-for-profit entity strictly supervised by the state, operating as an autonomous body governed by elected representatives of employers and employees. It defined healthcare financing as based on payroll contributions by employers and employees, set at 13.25 per cent of wages. The insurance contributions would be compulsory and constitute the basis of healthcare access.

The law also introduced patients' co-payment for medical goods and services. The benefit package of the compulsory insurance would cover a wide range of medical services, but most would be subject to cost-sharing, with patients' shares varying from 5 to more than 50 per cent of the service price. Patients would be exempt from making co-payments above a certain limit paid within a calendar year. The law did not include co-payment for emergency services or treatments for life-threatening conditions, and it exempted certain population groups, such as children and the elderly over the age of 75.

Co-payments were publicly perceived as highly controversial (Albreht 2011: 119). Even though co-payments (*participacija*) existed under socialism, they were low, and their increase in the post-communist context raised concerns about their impact on equal access to health services. A public opinion survey preceding the introduction of the 1992 law showed three quarters of Slovenians would be willing to contribute more of their financial resources to health if services were of higher quality, but only a minority—around 10 per cent—were ready to pay for health services directly from their own pocket (Toš 1991). World Bank experts were critical of co-payments as well, fearing the shifting of healthcare costs onto

[26] *Zakon o zdravstvenem varstvu in zdravstvenem zavarovanju—ZZVZZ*, Law no. 9/92.

patients could generate barriers to access for economically vulnerable populations.[27]

The government, however, justified its introduction of co-payments, arguing the main aim was to enhance private health expenditure, diversify expenditure sources and deflect the 'unnecessary' use of medical services (Albreht 2011: 119).

As it turned out, co-payment for health services was a topic of debate throughout the three transitional decades. However, after their introduction in the 1992 law, co-payments stayed in place despite the changes in the ideological orientation of the government and increased bipolarisation of party competition after 2004.[28] The first LDS government, as shown in the next section, insured this stability by introducing complementary private insurance as coverage for co-payments, thus confirming the shift towards healthcare financing as substantially dependent on private sources. The populist right-wing government led by Janez Janša (SDS) tried to reduce the public debate centred on equity issues by introducing exemptions for low-income groups in a 2008 amendment to the 1992 law.[29] Yet, this implied most Slovenians would still be obliged to pay for a part of their medical costs out of pocket to receive the needed care.

Co-payment became a major mechanism of the financial stability of the Slovenian health system, and this became evident during the 2008 global financial crisis. The country was hit hard by the crisis, experiencing rapidly worsening economic and labour market performances, a drop in GDP and an increase in unemployment rates (Guardiancich 2016). The 2011 elections, which took place in the midst of a crisis-driven economic downturn, were followed by the formation of a majority government by a right-leaning coalition led by the SDS and with Janša as Prime Minister. This government introduced a crisis law, the Law on Balancing Public Finances; notably, the law increased co-payments.[30] Even though this increase was partly mitigated by the reduction of prices for selected services introduced by the same law, co-payments remained the focus of public debate and,

[27] Interview No 1.

[28] The left-wing governments—LDS Drnovšek/Rop governments 1992–2004, SD Pahor government 2008–2012, PS Bratušek 2013–2014, and SMC Cerar government 2014–2018—left co-payments untouched.

[29] *Zakon o spremembah in dopolnitvah zakona o zdravstvenem varstvu in zdravstvenem zavarovanju*, Law no. 76/08.

[30] *Zakon za uravnoteženje javnih financ-ZUJF*, Law no. 40/12.

most importantly, justified the existence of another key market element of the country's health system—complementary private insurance.

Introduction of Complementary Private Insurance

Whilst the introduction of co-payments was the first step in the shift of the Slovenian health system towards private elements, a further step in this direction was taken with the introduction of complementary private insurance. An important political context was the emergence of the LDS as the dominant party in the country. Following the dissolution of the DEMOS coalition in spring 1992, LDS leader Janez Drnovšek took over Peterle's position of Prime Minister. The party's rise was confirmed in the December 1992 elections in which it won the majority of votes. The result was the formation of a centrist, left-liberal majority coalition government of the LDS and three other parties—the communist successor party (ZLSD), the left-leaning Slovenian Democratic Party (SDS), and the Christian Democrats (SKD). However, inter-coalitional conflicts led to re-arrangement of the government in April 1994; it remained under Drnovšek's leadership, but the coalition now included the LDS, the ZLSD and the SKD.

Governmental reshuffling notwithstanding, the continuity of health policy in this early transitional period was ensured by the stable leadership of Božidar Voljč as Minister of Health from 1992 to 1997. Voljč had been the head of the parliamentary Health Committee during Peterle's government which supported the introduction of co-payments, and he was personally in favour of a healthcare financing model that would involve both public insurance as obligatory and private health insurance as voluntary (see Voljč 1991). Therefore, when he became the Minister of Health, his Ministry proposed the introduction of voluntary health insurance, alongside the statutory health insurance; it would be used primarily as a complementary insurance covering co-payments. One of the core arguments was that voluntary health insurance would strengthen the plurality of healthcare financing sources. Another argument was that having the possibility to buy complementary health insurance would protect patients from potentially high healthcare costs generated by co-payments. This, it was argued, would resolve equity issues linked to co-payments (Cernić Istenić 1998; Albreht 2011).

In the amendment to the Law on Healthcare and Health Insurance,[31] voluntary private insurance was defined as insurance that could be offered to patients as a complement or supplement to the compulsory insurance. This insurance could cover partial costs of services covered by statutory insurance (i.e., co-payments), as well as costs of additional services not covered by the statutory insurance or costs of services of a higher standard. The law stipulated employers would be able to offer this voluntary insurance to their employees. The insurance would be managed by the Health Insurance Institute of Slovenia (HIIS), separately from the statutory insurance, but the law also said other insurance companies would be allowed to enter the voluntary health insurance market under equal conditions. The amendment clearly envisioned a competitive insurance market, stipulating that whilst the insurance companies must offer fixed premiums for a certain set of benefits, they could vary premiums for other benefits. Two insurance companies entered the market for voluntary health insurance shortly thereafter. One was HIIS, as non-for-profit public insurance company, which according to the amendment, was legally obliged to offer voluntary health insurance and the other was Adriatic Slovenica, a private for-profit insurance company.

Private health insurance met with significant success, but also had problems. A large majority of the Slovenian population bought complementary insurance to cover co-payments (Milenković Kramer 2009; Albreht 2011), with private spending for healthcare reaching 13.5 per cent by 2000 (Albreht et al. 2002), and the CPI started being considered quasi-obligatory.[32] There were several issues, however. One was the burden of premiums. Voluntary insurance initially implied that employees did not cover their premiums; rather, these were covered by their employers. This was seen as problematic, especially in the public sector, and led to a court case in which the Slovenian Court of Accounts found the employer's payment of private insurance for employees in a public sector was against the principle of the solid management of public funds (Court of Accounts 1996). As a result, public sector employees had to start paying their own premiums (Albreht 2011: 119). This, in turn, raised issues of inequality, as the premiums of the privately employed continued to be covered by their employers.

[31] *Zakon o spremembah in dopolnitvah zakona o zdravstvenem varstvu in zdravstvenem zavarovanju—ZZVZZ-A*, Law no. 13/93.

[32] Interview No. 4.

Another issue was that voluntary insurance became practically compulsory for individuals with chronic illnesses, as otherwise, they risked significant medical costs (Albreht 2011: 130). There were also institutional issues centred on the relationship between the two insurance types within the HIIS. As defined by the 1993 amendment, the HIIS was legally obliged to provide voluntary insurance, and it soon became the largest provider of voluntary health insurance (Albreht et al. 2002). This raised concerns that compulsory and voluntary insurance should be administered separately. An additional criticism of voluntary insurance was that the introduction of complementary insurance made co-payments ineffective, as it did not deter patients from seeking unnecessary care—the government's argument for the introduction of co-payments in the first place (Albreht et al. 2009).

Even though multiple problems were generated by the introduction of voluntary insurance, thanks to the stable political context, the government was able to resolve some of the policy deficiencies, adapting the voluntary health insurance to the existing context of healthcare provision. In 1998, under another LDS-led coalition government, Parliament amended the 1993 law separating the voluntary tier from the obligatory health insurance tier, stipulating that a new insurance company called Vzajemna would be established independently of the HIIS as a mutual not-for-profit health insurance company (Albreht et al. 2002).[33]

First Attempt to Abolish Complementary Private Insurance

Although numerous problems arose with the introduction of complementary private insurance, it was only at the beginning of the second transitional decade that more concrete moves towards its abolition took place. Interestingly, this happened under a government still led by the LDS, who was responsible for its introduction. After its victory in the 2000 elections, the LDS formed a government with the communist successor party (ZLSD) and two other parties, the Slovenian People Party (SPP) and the Democratic Party of Pensioners of Slovenia (DeSUS). Initially led by Drnovšek, the government leadership was taken over by Anton Rop in 2002, with Dušan Keber (*LDS*) as Minister of Health. Keber's Ministry initiated a debate on the reform of the health system in 2003, publishing

[33] *Zakon o spremembah in dopolnitvah zakona o zdravstvenem varstvu in zdravstvenem zavarovanju—ZZVZZ-C*, Law no. 29/98.

a White Paper titled *Health Reform* (Ministry of Health 2003; see also Keber et al. 2003; Keber 2003).

The reform document, authored by Keber and a group of healthcare experts, argued the healthcare system should be reformed, putting an emphasis on fairness in allocating healthcare funds, distributing care according to needs, improving healthcare access and more effectively regulating the system as a whole. To this end, it put forward a comprehensive reform plan, the main element of which was the abolition of complementary private insurance. Building on the already controversial topic of private insurance, the document criticised the reform of the 1990s, interpreting the introduction of complementary private insurance as a part of a carefully planned withdrawal of public funding. It noted that all holders of voluntary insurance had to pay the same premium, thus making it regressive and eroding the solidarity of the population.[34] It proposed merging complementary insurance, which was almost universal, with compulsory insurance (Keber et al. 2003).

The Ministry's reform proposal soon generated disagreement. Interestingly, the proposal came from inside the LDS and when it was first presented, lacked support within the government and amongst party ranks. The proposal was also strongly opposed by the Minister of Finance Dušan Mramor, who argued the abolition of complementary private insurance by merging it with compulsory insurance was unfeasible; it would inevitably lead to an increase in compulsory insurance contributions, and this, in turn, would lead to an increase in labour costs.[35] The Ministry of Finance even commissioned a special review of the proposal; it concluded that whilst the Ministry of Health's proposal provided a good basis for the start of the reform process, it lacked clarity. The review stressed the need to consider fiscal implications and, more importantly, other reform options.[36]

In its attempt to gain the support of social partners, the Ministry of Health presented the outline of the healthcare reform plan to the Economic and Social Council, the tripartite body in charge of social dialogue, and to the National Council, the Upper House of Parliament. The proposal, however, had a negative reception, as both trade unions and the employers' organisation representatives opposed it, arguing the merging of

[34] Interviews No. 3 and 5.

[35] Interviews No. 1, 6 and 7.

[36] Interview No. 4.

voluntary and compulsory insurance would lead to an increase in compulsory contributions (National Council 2003). The trade union of doctors was another main source of opposition, vocally criticising the reform and calling the Ministry's proposal 'an eggshell without content' (RTVSLO 2003). Unsurprisingly, the insurance companies also expressed their opposition to the abolition of voluntary insurance (Milenković Kramer 2009; Albreht et al. 2016). This widespread criticism was used by the government to argue that the Ministry's reform proposals for the abolition of complementary private insurance lacked the support of the main stakeholders and should be abandoned. As a consequence, the proposal never reached parliamentary procedure.

Adaptation of Complementary Private Insurance

Issues with complementary private insurance persisted, with new issues emerging over time. In the early 2000s, the voluntary insurance market began to voice significant concerns, generating textbook examples of market failures in healthcare provision. The high demand for complementary private insurance led to the expansion of the insurance market so that beside Adriatic Slovenica and Vzajemna, other two insurance companies, Triglav and Merkur, started offering complementary private insurance. This led to cream-skimming, as these companies launched campaigns aimed at younger and healthier individuals, offering risk-related premiums (Calcoen and van de Ven 2017).

These new problems coincided with the end of LDS's decade-plus leadership in Slovenian politics. The right-wing SDS was victorious in the 2004 elections; together with three other parties (NSi, SLS and DeSUS), it formed a right-wing majority government under Janez Janša. To solve the cream-skimming problem, in 2005, Janša's government launched an amendment to the 1992 Law on Healthcare and Health Insurance. The amendment introduced a risk adjustment scheme to level out differences between insurance companies in terms of healthcare costs. It stipulated all insurance companies must apply a unified flat premium irrespective of premium holders' sex, age or health status, and it introduced supervision of the insurance market, whereby insurance companies had to provide financial reports quarterly to the Ministry of Health.[37]

[37] *Zakon o spremembah in dopolnitvah zakona o zdravstvenem varstvu in zdravstvenem zavarovanju- ZZVZZ-UPB2*, Law no. 09/05.

In addition, the amendment introduced tighter regulation of voluntary health insurance. This aspect of the amendment became highly controversial. The amendment stipulated, for example, that if foreign health insurance companies wished to enter the country's voluntary health insurance market, they had to establish a branch office in Slovenia. The most controversial aspect, however, was the amendment's specification of a set of controls on private health insurance companies over issues such as the companies' use of profit and prior approval of premium increases. Companies had to gain approval for an increase in premiums from the Ministry of Health, and the reserves from the profit generated by voluntary insurance schemes could not be transferred into the capital of insurance companies.[38]

These provisions, unsurprisingly, triggered fierce criticism from the insurance companies, who turned to the European Commission for an opinion on the conformity of the 2005 amendment to EU law. In 2007, the Commission sent a letter of formal notice to Slovenia stating certain articles of the contested amendment breached EU directives on non-life insurance. In response, the Slovenian government argued that although complementary health insurance was not compulsory, it was part of the country's social insurance system, as it represented a matter of public interest. The discussion between the government and the Commission became protracted, with the former showing little willingness to change the problematic provisions. The Commission referred the case to the European Court of Justice (Calcoen and van de Ven 2017). In 2012, the Court concluded the provisions of the 2005 amendment breached the EU regulations on competition and free movement of capital and asked Slovenia to repeal the provisions to avoid hindering the operation of a free market (European Court of Justice 2012; see also Calcoen and van de Ven 2017). The contested provisions were subsequently removed, demonstrating both the power of selective corporatism and its limits in the broader supranational context.

Janša's government introduced another important change in a special law related to the status of the only non-profit insurance company, Vzajemna. The 2007 Law on Conditions for Status Transforming of Vzajemna envisaged that the company would be restructured as a joint stock company, thus redefining its clients as members and owners of the

[38] Law no. 09/05.

company.[39] This law was opposed by Vzajemna itself, but both the ZLSD, now renamed the Social Democrats (SD), and the LDS supported it (Delo 2007). The National Council also opposed the law, arguing that keeping Vzajemna's existing status was a matter of public interest and an issue of large financial resources. The Council stressed that in the context of EU membership, 'Slovenia should support the establishment of non-profit organisations with a social goal, which would operate on the democratic principle of members, users and employees and be based on the solidarity of its members' (National Council 2007). The Lower House passed the law without a vote against it (National Assembly 2007), once again demonstrating the strong party consensus on the direction of health policy.

This party consensus was soon challenged, however. Janša's government introduced a proposal for the Amendment of the Law on Ownership Restructuring of Insurance Companies. The proposal envisaged further privatisation of the country's largest insurance company, Triglav, by allowing one of shareholders, Kapitalska Družba, to sell its shares. Arguing against this amendment after it was passed in Parliament, the members of the National Council decided to send it to a national referendum on 11 November 2007. In the referendum, 71 per cent of citizens voted against the proposed amendment. Therefore, Triglav's shares could not be sold or divided amongst former policy holders (see Štrus 2019). The fact that the National Council prevented further privatisation of Triglav illustrates the limits of the party consensus and institutional influence on the policymaking process. Yet, this policy episode also provides support for the case of selective corporatism, as parties sided with insurance companies to keep complementary private insurance in place (under Keber) and fostered further privatisation of the insurance sector, but also introduced controls on the profit-making of the insurance companies—even though these were later withdrawn after the intervention of the European Court of Justice.

Second Attempt to Abolish Complementary Private Insurance

The 2008 elections resulted in the victory of the Social Democrats (SD, former ZLSD). The SD formed a centre-left majority government with its old government partner LDS, the pensioner's party (DeSUS) and the social-liberal party (ZARES) under Borut Pahor. This government led Slovenia at the beginning of the economic and financial crisis. The effects

[39] *Zakon o pogojih za statusno preoblikovanje Vzajemne zdravstvene zavarovalnice d.v.z.—ZPSPVZZ*, Law no. 60/07.

were felt in 2009, with a drop in GDP and dramatically increasing unemployment.

In 2011, the Pahor government outlined a reform plan for healthcare, titled 'Healthcare System Upgrade until 2020—Step Ahead' (Ministry of Health 2011). The plan included a wide set of reform measures, including a redefinition of the basic benefit package, but its most radical proposal was to abolish complementary private insurance. This proposal drew on the 2003 White Paper, as it criticised the lack of solidarity in the existing scheme, but it proposed a different plan. Complementary private insurance should be eliminated by providing the necessary funds from public resources, either by increasing the contribution rate for employees by two percentage points, or by covering the difference directly from the budget (Ministry of Health 2011; see also Stanovnik and Turk 2011).

Like the 2003 proposal, this one never reached parliamentary procedure. The Ministry's reform plan was not supported by the government and was caught up in a political debate. Parties of the government said that in principle they supported the abolition, but they questioned the feasibility of its implementation, especially in the context of the financial crisis (Delo 2011). The plan was additionally thwarted by the upcoming elections that led to the change of government (Stanovnik and Prevolnik-Rupel 2014).

The context of the financial crisis allowed further growth of private insurance in Slovenian healthcare. In September 2011, Pahor's government fell after a vote of no confidence; after an election, a new government was formed as a majority right-leaning coalition of SDS and four other parties (DeSUS, Nsi-KLS, SLS, and DL), again under Janša. This government introduced a crisis law, the Law on Balancing Public Finances, which increased co-payments for health services.[40] Even though this increase was partly mitigated by the reduction of prices for selected services, complementary private insurance premiums increased, and this, in turn, led to a growth in the private health spending share of the total healthcare expenditure (Milenković Kramer 2016; Albreht et al. 2016). As one of the country's health experts saw it, the increase in co-payments was justified by the general view that without complementary private insurance, the crisis in health would never end.[41] Even so, co-payments and complementary private insurance remained topics of public debate in the

[40] *Zakon za uravnoteženje javnih financ-ZUJF*, Law no. 40/12.

[41] Interview No. 1.

aftermath of the financial crisis. The share of private healthcare spending reached 27.3 per cent of the country's total health expenditure on health in 2019 (OECD 2019).

Limited Privatisation of Primary Care

Another key reform debate in the Slovenian context, beyond co-payments and complementary insurance, concerned the privatisation of primary care. Similar to the discussions on healthcare financing, this debate was initiated in early transition and showed a clear vision based on a gradual rather than a radical approach to policy change. Unlike healthcare financing, however, the reform of primary care was based on a predominantly public model of service provision.

The general debate on whether delivery of healthcare services should be kept public or handed over to the private sector was initiated under the early transitional Peterle's government. The dominant view of experts, as well as those within the government, was that primary care in the new healthcare system could allow some privatisation, but this type of care should substantially build on the existing model's network of public community health centres. This model dated back to the interwar period and was based on the ideas of social medicine promoted by Andrija Štampar. In the context of the post-communist reform debate, this system was recognised as a strong feature of the old socialist healthcare model, supporting the view that primary care should essentially be kept in public hands.[42]

In addition, privatisation of the public community health centres was seen as problematic from the point of view of coordination and supervision of healthcare delivery. As argued by Božidar Voljč, head of the parliamentary Health Committee under Peterle's government, privatisation should not be opposed in principle, but reformers should be warned that the introduction of private delivery carried different types of risks (Voljč 1991). More specifically, privatisation and competition between public and private providers risked the establishment of two unrelated systems of healthcare service delivery, might prevent supervision and lead to the ongoing taxation of private healthcare. Voljč's biggest concern, however, was the impact of privatisation on the existing organisation of primary care and a potential increase in the number of doctors. He also warned of the sharp separation between primary and secondary care, arguing that in practice,

[42] Interview No. 3.

this would mean a longer referral chain, and this, in turn, risked duplication of examinations and equipment (Voljč 1991).

Voljč's views were a reflection of the more general view expressed in health policy circles according to which healthcare delivery could be privatised, but at the same time, the privatisation should be controlled and heavily regulated process (Cernič Istenič 1998). This was linked to another generally accepted view that private delivery should be allowed only if the publicly delivered primary care could not satisfy the population's health needs. The decision to opt for a controlled and heavily regulated privatisation process was built on a political consensus, which was so strong that the government did not allow the involvement of foreign experts with potentially opposing views and even ignored privatisation demands from those healthcare professionals who favoured it.[43]

Healthcare professionals, whose interests were still not represented by the professional chambers,[44] expressed their opposition and engaged in a fervent debate with the government. The main issue was the government's plan to keep the public and private sectors separate by establishing that healthcare professionals could not work in the public and private sectors at the same time. The professionals opposed this provision, arguing it would make the opening of private practice much more difficult, turning it into a risky endeavour. A combination of public and private involvement, they said, would help the privatisation process, as it would allow the gradual acquisition of patients, resources and equipment, and make the opening of private practice much easier. The Ministry of Health rejected this argument, claiming the public–private mix was not recommended by the World Health Organisation; the two sectors had to be kept separate because the main purpose of privatisation was to promote competition and reduce unemployment of healthcare workers (Cernič Istenič 1998).

Unsurprisingly, it was under Drnovšek's government with Voljč as Minister of Health, that Parliament passed the 1992 Law on Healthcare Services allowing heavily regulated privatisation of primary care.[45] This law introduced privatisation at the municipal level. It stipulated the privatisation process would be based on the strict principle that permission for private practice in the existing public system should not lead to an increase in the overall provision of healthcare services, and these permissions

[43] Interviews No. 1 and 2.

[44] The Slovenian Medical Chamber was re-established in 1992.

[45] *Zakon o zdravstveni dejavnosti—ZZDej*, Law No. 9/92.

should take local health needs and capacities into consideration. The opening of private practice was to be organised on the basis of concessions, and priority was to be given to doctors who leased consulting rooms in public health facilities. This implied that rather than exercising their private practice independently, healthcare professionals would be given a concession to deliver healthcare as a public service. If the concessionaries failed to deliver this service in conformity with the laws and regulations, their concession could be taken away by the Ministry of Health. Overall, this reflected a highly regulated privatisation process in which privatisation was managed at the local level but implemented under the strict control of the state.[46]

With respect to the combination of public and private work, the 1992 Law on Health Services suggested some level of compromise with healthcare professionals' demands. It envisaged doctors working in the public sector would be able to treat private patients in their domiciliary community health centres and be paid for these private services through out-of-pocket payments.[47] This provision did not satisfy professionals' expectations, however, as it did not establish clear rules according to which this type of private provision would work in practice. Consequently, the debate over the public–private work mix continued (Cernić Istenić 1998).

The highly regulated model of privatisation introduced in the 1992 law led to a relatively slow privatisation process. By 1995, only 10 per cent of all doctors in Slovenia were registered as self-employed (Hočevar 1996; see also Švab et al. 2001). An issue that remained a focus of the policy debate over the coming decades was the privatisation model based on concessions. Procedures for granting concessions continued to be criticised by doctors as ambiguous and, in their view, were responsible for low privatisation rates. Yet, as privatisation of primary care in Slovenia was simply 'not politically feasible', this led to the continued opposition of the government to the demands of healthcare professionals for the expanded privatisation of healthcare delivery.[48]

The debate over the public–private dimension of healthcare delivery was exacerbated by an emerging discussion on patient rights. The 1992 Law on Healthcare and Health Insurance defined one of these rights as

[46] Interview No. 1.
[47] Law No. 9/92.
[48] Interview No. 7.

the right to freely choose one's doctor,[49] but problematically, this right could be applied only to doctors working in the public sector. In 1997, a group of doctors filed a claim, asking the Constitutional Court to check the constitutionality of this rule. The Court determined a patient's right applied equally to public and private doctors (Slovenian Constitutional Court 1998).

The rules clarifying the privatisation process based on concessions finally became less ambiguous—a decade after the introduction of the 1992 Law on Health Services. The 2004 amendment, introduced by Janša's right-wing government, provided a clearer definition of the process of granting concessions, specified the limitations and validity of the concessions and introduced the concept of free specialists.[50] Whilst this amendment was seen as opening opportunities for further privatisation of healthcare delivery, a counter movement, 'Movement for the Preservation of Public Health' (*Gibanje za Ohranitev Javnega Zdravstva*), criticised the privatisation process, arguing it involved uncontrolled and non-transparent concessions. This movement, led by representatives of the Trade Union of Health and Social Welfare (*Sindikat Zdravstva in Socialnega Varstva Slovenije*), advocated the need for the defence of the public system against the government's privatisation. It contended politicians should recognise solidarity as a deeply rooted value of the Slovenian health system and stressed the need for health services to be equally accessible to all citizens (Ohranimo 2006). Minister of Health Andrej Bručan tried to buffer the government from criticism by claiming that granting concessions in healthcare was not the same as privatising healthcare (Javornik 2006) and by arguing against accusations of 'wild privatisation' (RTVSLO 2006).

New attempts to regulate and restrict the privatisation process, also contributing to the polarisation of views over policy direction, appeared under Pahor's left-wing government. In 2009, Pahor's government put forward a draft for a new Law on Health Services. The draft suggested a stricter tendering procedure and procurement rules for the commissioning of services from private providers reimbursed from public funds. Another provision was a decrease in the influence of professional associations, with the draft proposing abolition of mandatory membership in professional chambers (Ministry of Health 2009). As these provisions

[49] *Zakon o zdravstvenem varstvu in zdravstvenem zavarovanju—ZZVZZ*, Law no. 9/92.

[50] *Zakon o spremembah in dopolnitvah zakona o zdravstveni dejavnosti—ZZDej-G*, Law No. 2/04.

went against healthcare professionals' interests and aimed at curtailing their power, once it was presented for public debate, the draft unsurprisingly faced fierce criticism. Professionals argued the intended law would diminish the role of private practice and representatives of the medical, pharmacist and nursing chambers argued non-mandatory memberships could lead to several competing chambers. The medical chamber disagreed with other provisions of the draft, for example, the stipulation of a state-controlled process determining posts for doctors' specialty training and the establishment of a state-run institute for healthcare quality. The draft met with only moderate approval within the governing coalition (SD, DeSUS, ZARES, and LDS), and as a result, it never entered the parliamentary procedure (Albreht 2009a, 2009b).

The issue of private healthcare delivery and the public–private work mix remained a hot topic during the third post-communist decade. In 2013, the left-wing government under Miro Cerar proposed another amendment to the 1992 Law on Healthcare Services; this one aimed at restricting both privatisation and the public–private mix. The debate on this proposal featured the strong and fervent opposition of healthcare professionals and became protracted when a civil society organisation, the Society for the Health of the Nation (*Društvo za zdravje naroda*), tried to call for a national referendum and failed (RTVSLO 2017). In spite of the opposition, the government finally adopted the amendment in 2017.[51]

The new legislation defined health services delivered in the public sector as public services, thus implying they were non-commercial and not-for-profit activities. It also introduced more transparent procedures for granting concessions to private healthcare providers. In addition, profits from delivery of healthcare services through concessions must be reinvested in public healthcare provision and service development, with these services defined as 'non-commercial services of general interest'. Finally, the amendment regulated the work of healthcare professionals outside their employing institutions, allowing work in other structures, but under very strict conditions (Ministry of Health 2017; Albreht et al. 2021).

Resorting to the Constitutional Court, the Association of Private Doctors and Dentists and the Medical Chamber questioned the constitutionality of the amendment. Arguing the provisions limited economic

[51] *Zakon o spremembah in dopolnitvah zakona o zdravstvenem varstvu in zdravstvenem zavarovanju*, Law no. 64/17.

freedom, they asked the Court to consider those provisions that changed conditions for obtaining and revoking licences to perform healthcare activities, tightened the granting of concessions, and restricted private healthcare activities by stipulating the concessionaries' profits generated from healthcare delivery be reinvested in the development of public healthcare (RTVSLO 2018). The Court decided against most of the professionals' claims, stating parts of the law regulating licences and tightening concessions were in accordance with the Constitution. However, it also decided the amendment's provisions limiting the use of financial surpluses generated by the concessionaries should be repealed. It justified this decision by arguing that restricting the freedom to dispose of surplus revenues limited the entrepreneurial freedom of private individuals, interfered with their economic initiative and undermined one of the key motivations for performing the concessional activity (Slovenian Constitutional Court 2018).

The repeal of parts of the 2017 amendment was certainly a victory for health professionals, pointing to the limits of the government's power to circumscribe professional influence on policymaking. The judgement of the Constitutional Court in favour of the ability of concessionaries to retain profit from their activities was clearly motivated by the 2011 decision of the European Court of Justice; on the basis of EU law, it had similarly decided in favour of the insurance companies, allowing them to retain their profits. In fact, the Court related its decision to EU law, arguing that not being allowed to determine 'how to allocate the surplus of revenue over expenditure very significantly narrows the scope of entrepreneurial freedom of private providers and interferes with their economic initiative' (Slovenian Constitutional Court 2018). Despite this victory in the professionals' camp, however, privatisation of Slovenian healthcare delivery remained severely limited because of the highly controlled process of granting concessions.

Lack of Hospital Privatisation

A final key policy issue in the context of Slovenian's post-communist healthcare developments was hospital privatisation. Hospital privatisation, or rather, the lack thereof, demonstrates the sturdy character of the country's particular public–private healthcare mix. In sharp contrast to the privatisation of primary care, the privatisation of public hospitals was never hotly debated. During the privatisation debates in the early transition, the main discussions revolved around issue of primary care. In fact, the transformation of hospitals into private entities was not even considered a policy option. A dominant view in this period was that public hospitals, particular those in bigger cities, were relatively large organisations consuming a significant portion of public healthcare spending. Therefore, it was not in the state's best interests to privatise hospitals.[52]

The view that Slovenian hospitals should remain in public hands predominated in policy circles over the following decades despite the growing problem of considerable hospital debt. With the 2008 global financial crisis, hospital debt became a main issue in health policy debate, as the majority of public hospitals recorded losses. Instead of proposing ownership change, however, one policy proposal was that hospitals should cover these losses by taking loans from the government. This idea was abandoned, as it was not clear how these loans could be repaid (Stanovnik and Prevolnik-Rupel 2014).

The problem of hospital debts grew in the aftermath of the global crisis. In 2016, a group of 15 insolvent hospitals recorded 170 million EUR debt (Jovanović 2020). The insolvency issues also created obstacles in the day-to-day functioning of the hospital sector, causing problems such as lack of materials and medicines, delayed payments of salaries and increasing waiting times, at the time, a major issue in patients' access to services (Jovanović 2020; see also Prevolnik-Rupel 2018).

In 2017, one of the smallest opposition parties, the Christian Democrat New Slovenia (*Nova Slovenia—NSi*), proposed an emergency meeting of the parliamentary Health Committee. In their statement, the party members underlined the huge hospital losses, arguing a core problem was the state dominance of the hospital sector. The state, they said, was the client, the payer and the regulator of services. They suggested abolishing the state monopoly by handing over certain hospitals to private institutions in the form of private projects (Nova Slovenia 2017). Yet, this vision did not become a concrete policy proposal, as it ran against the government's view of the problem and its solution.

The government's solution for the hospital debt problem was revealed in the autumn of 2017 when Miro Cerar's government introduced a special law outlining a recovery plan for public hospitals, whereby their debts

[52] Interview No. 1.

would be covered by the state budget.[53] As a consequence, the 15 hospitals mentioned above received 136 million EUR, covering 80 per cent of the debt (*Insajder* 2018). The end result was that the large majority of Slovenian hospitals remained in public hands (Albreht et al. 2021).

Conclusion

This chapter has accounted for the development of the healthcare policy model in post-communist Slovenia, an intriguing public–private mix in which medical services are delivered almost exclusively through healthcare facilities in public ownership, but the financing of these services is essentially reliant on a market instrument—complementary private insurance. It analysed the key policy episodes that contributed to driving the development of this peculiar policy model and accounted for its shaping factors. It suggested the market-oriented policy experiences under socialism, consensual politics of the early transition and the institutional configuration with few vetoes were key factors in the establishment of this policy model through a relatively smooth process of policy learning. The combination of these factors contributed to path-dependent policy development; this, in turn, allowed the gradual adaptation of market-oriented ideas and resulted in the *survival* of market reforms over time—in stark contrast to the Czech experience of *instability* and the Polish *reversal*.

References

Albreht, Tit. 2009a. Public debate on Health Services Act proposal ends. Accessed 10 June 2021. http://www.hpm.org/survey/si/a14/4.

———. 2009b. New health reform start. Accessed 10 June 2021. http://www.hpm.org/survey/si/a13/4.

———. 2011. *Slovenian health care in transition: Studies on the changes in the Slovenian health care system from 1985 until 2010*. PhD Thesis, University of Amsterdam. Accessed 15 June 2021 https://pure.uva.nl/ws/files/1405936/85921_thesis.pdf.

Albreht, Tit, and Niek Klazinga. 2009. Privatisation of health care in Slovenia in the period 1992–2008. *Health Policy* 90 (2–3): 262–269.

Albreht, Tit, Marjan Cesen, Elke Jakubowski, Boris Kramberger, Malden Markota, Vesna Kerstin Petrič, Marjan Premik, and Martin Toth. 2002. *Healthcare sys-*

[53] *Zakon o interventnih ukrepih za zagotovitev finančne stabilnosti javnih zdravstvenih zavodov, katerih ustanovitelj je Republika Slovenija—ZIUFSZZ*, Law no. 54/17.

tems in transition: Slovenia. European Observatory on Healthcare Systems and Policies. WHO.

Albreht, Tit, Eva Turk, Martin Toth, Jakov Ceglar, Stane Marn, Radivoje Pribaković-Brnovec, and Marco Schäfer. 2009. *Health care systems in transition: Slovenia*. European Observatory on Healthcare Systems and Policies. WHO.

Albreht, Tit, Radivoje Pribaković Brinovec, Dušan Jošar, Mircha Poldrugovac Tatjana Kostnapfel, Metka Zaletel, Dimitra Panteli, and Anna Maresso. 2016. *Health care systems in transition: Slovenia*. European Observatory on Healthcare Systems and Policies. WHO.

Albreht, Tit, K. Polin, Radivoje P. Brinovec, Marjeta Kuhar, Mircha Poldrugovac, Petra O. Rehberger, Valentina Prevolnik-Rupel, and Pia Vracko. 2021. *Health care systems in transition: Slovenia*. European Observatory on Healthcare Systems and Policies. WHO.

Barr, Nicholas A. 1994. *Labor markets and social policy in Central and Eastern Europe: The transition and beyond*. Washington, DC: World Bank Publications.

Berg, Robert L., Roy M. Brooks, and Miomir Savićević. 1976. *Health care in Yugoslavia and the United States*. Bethesda: National Institute of Health.

Boh Katja. 1989. Prispevek k poskusom za prestrukturiranje zdravstva. In *Prestrukturiranje družbenih dejavnosti*, ed. I. Svetlik, 20–25. Ljubljana: Raziskovalno Poročilo ISU.

Brown, Theodeore M., and Elisabeth Fee. 2006. Andrija Štampar: Charismatic leader of social medicine and international health. *American Journal of Public Health* 96 (8): 1383.

Brus Alojz. 1990. Odprta vprašanja novega zakona o zdravstvenem varstvu. *Zdravstveni Vestnik* 6: 301–308.

Bugajski, Janusz. 2002. *Political parties of Eastern Europe: A guide to politics in the post-communist era*. Armonk, New York, and London: Sharpe.

Cabada, Ladislav. 2005. Slovenian united list of social democrats: Post-communist or post-modern political party? In *Trajectories of the left social democratic and (ex) communist parties in contemporary Europe: Between past and future*, ed. L. Kopeček, 150–164. Prague: Charles University Prague.

Calcoen, Piet, and Wynand P. van de Ven. 2017. Voluntary additional health insurance in the European Union: Free market or regulation? *European Journal of Health Law* 24 (5): 591–613.

Cernić Istenić, Majda. 1998. Privatization of health care in Slovenia. *Croatian Medical Journal* 39: 288–297.

Constitution of the Republic of Slovenia. 1991. Accessed 2 June 2021. http://www.us-rs.si/legal-basis/constitution/?lang=en.

Court of Accounts. 1996. *Poročilo o delu Računskega sodišča od* 1.1.1995 do 31.3.1996, št.3105-1/96-2. *Računsko sodišče Republike Slovenije*, Ljubljana, 8.5.1996, pp. 5-9-5-11.

Delo. 2007. *Zakon za morebitno preoblikovanje vzajemne* [Law on the possible transformation of Vzajemna]. Accessed 4 August 2021. https://old.delo.si/novice/slovenija/zakon-za-morebitno-preoblikovanje-vzajemne.html.
———. 2011. *Za ukinitev prostovoljnega zavarovanja vecina strank* [Most parties for abolition of voluntary health insurance]. Accessed 8 August 2021. https://old.delo.si/novice/politika/za-ukinitev-prostovoljnega-zavarovanja-vecina-strank.html.
Dobaja, Dunja. 2009. Zdravstveno in socialno varstvo v Sloveniji v letih 1945–1953 s poudarkom na razvoju zakonodaje. *Prispevki za novejšo zgodovino* 2: 125–147.
Estrin, Saul. 1991. Yugoslavia: The case of self-managing market socialism. *Journal of Economic Perspectives* 5 (4): 187–194.
European Court of Justice. 2012. Case C-185/11, Commission v. Slovenia, 26 January 2012. Accessed 13 August 2021. https://op.europa.eu/en/publication-detail/-/publication/032b235c-db43-47ec-beed-5ecda2cb255e/language-en.
Fasone, Christina. 2019. Concluding chapter: Unicameralism and masked bicameralism. In *Constitutional reform of national legislatures*, ed. L. Albert, A. Barragia, and C. Fasone, 183–192. Cheltenham: Edward Elgar Publishing.
Field, Mark. 1989. *Success and crisis in national health systems.* New York: Routledge.
Fink-Hafner, Danica. 1998. Organized interests in the policy-making process in Slovenia. *Journal of European Public Policy* 5 (2): 285–302.
———. 2006. Slovenia: Between bipolarity and broad coalition-building. In *Post-communist EU member states: Parties and party systems*, ed. S. Jungerstam-Mulders, 203–231. Aldershot, Burlington: Ashgate.
———. 2019. Slovenia after 1989. In *Central and Southeast European politics since 1989*, ed. S.P. Ramet and C.M. Hassenstab. Cambridge and New York: Cambridge University Press.
Fink-Hafner, Danica, and Alenka Krašovec. 2005. Is consultation everything? The influence of interest groups on parliamentary working bodies in Slovenia. *Czech Sociological Review* 41 (3): 401–422.
Guardiancich, Igor. 2012. *Pension reforms in Central, Eastern and Southeastern Europe: From post-socialist transition to the global financial crisis.* Oxfordshire: Routledge.
———. 2016. Slovenia: The end of a success story? When a partial reform equilibrium turns bad. *Europe-Asia Studies* 68 (2): 205–231.
Himmelstein, David U., Slobodan Lang, and Steffie Woolhandler. 1984. The Yugoslav health system: Public ownership and local control. *Journal of Public Health Policy* 5 (3): 423–431.
Hočevar, Zdravko. 1996. *Health care systems in transition: Slovenia.* European Observatory on Healthcare Systems and Policies. WHO.

Hrast, Maša F., Ellen M. Immergut, Tatjana Rakar, Urban Boljka, Diana Burlacu, and Andra Roescu. 2018. Healthcare futures: Visions of solidarity and the sustainability of European healthcare systems. In *Attitudes, aspirations and welfare*, ed. P. Taylor-Gooby and B. Leruth, 215–242. London: Palgrave Macmillan.

Immergut, Ellen M. 1990. Institutions, veto points, and policy results: A comparative analysis of health care. *Journal of Public Policy* 10 (4): 391–416.

Insajder. 2018. *Bolnišnice morajo do konca marca pripraviti sanacijske programe* [Hospitals must prepare rehabilitation programmes by the end of March]. Accessed 10 August 2021. https://insajder.com/slovenija/bolnisnice-morajo-do-konca-marca-pripraviti-sanacijske-programe.

Janko Lojze. 1990. Kako do primernih sredstev za zdravstvo, šolstvo, kulturo. *Zdravstveni vestnik* 9: 290–297.

Javornik, Lojze. 2006. *Privatizacije v zdravstvu ni, pravi minister Bručan* [There is no privatisation in healthcare, says minister Bručan]. Accessed 10 August 2021. https://www.finance.si/170435/Privatizacije-v-zdravstvu-ni-pravi-minister-Brucan.

Jošt-Doma, Anka. 1983. *Participacija v zdravstvu. Naša Skupnost* 4.

Jovanović, Tatjana. 2020. Challenges of the Slovenian healthcare system exposed in hospitals' recovery plans. In *The importance of health informatics in public health during a pandemic*, ed. J. Mantas, A. Hasman, and M.S. Househ, 354–358. Amsterdam, Berlin, and Washington: IOS Press.

Keber, Dušan. 2003. *Utrjevanje vrednot in vzpodbujanje sprememb: Zdravstvena reforma* 2003 [Strengthening values and encouraging changes: Health reform 2003]. *Zdravstveni Vestnik* 73: 57–58.

Keber, Dušan, Tit Albreht, Polona Brčar, Silva Pečar-Čad, Irena Kirar-Fazarinc, and Mladen Markota. 2003. *Health reform—A draft*. Ljubljana: Ministry of Health of the Republic of Slovenia.

Komadina, Dominik. 1988. *Kako ozdraviti zdravstvo? Zdravstveno Varstvo* 27 (6/8): 201–209.

Krašovec, Alenka, and Tim Haughton. 2011. Money, organization and the state: The partial cartelization of party politics in Slovenia. *Communist and Post-Communist Studies* 44 (3): 199–209.

Krašovec, Alenka, and Lars Johannsen. 2016. Recent developments in democracy in Slovenia. *Problems of Post-Communism* 63 (5-6): 313–322.

Kunitz, Stephen J. 1979. Health care and workers' self-management in Yugoslavia. *International Journal of Health Services* 9(3): 521–537.

Lindstrom, Nicole, and Dóra Piroska. 2004. *The Politics of Europeanization in Europe's Southeastern Periphery: Slovenian Banks and Breweries on S(c)ale*. Queens' Papers on Europeanisation, No. p0045. Queens University Belfast.

Lukšić, Igor. 2003. Corporatism packaged in pluralist ideology: The case of Slovenia. *Communist and Post-Communist Studies* 36 (4): 509–525.

Markota, Mladen, and Tit Albreht. 2001. Slovenian experience on health insurance (re) introduction. *Croatian Medical Journal* 42 (1): 18–23.

Milanović, Vladimir, and Vuk Stambolović. 1985. The prescription for Yugoslav medicine. *Social Science and Medicine* 21 (7): 730–732.

Milenković Kramer, Anja. 2009. Slovenia. In *Private health insurance in the European Union*, ed. S. Thomson and E. Mossialos, 295–309. Brussels: European Commission.

———. 2016. Slovenia. In *Voluntary health insurance in Europe: Country experience*, ed. A. Sagan and S. Thomson, 133–139. World Health Organization.

Ministry of Health. 2003. *Zdravstvena reforma. Pravičnost, dostopnost, kakovost, učinkovitost* [Health reform: justice, accessibility, quality, efficiency]. Ljubljana: Ministry of Health.

———. 2009. *Javna razprava zakona o zdravstveni dejavnosti* [Public debate on the law on healthcare activity]. Accessed 2 August 2021. http://www.mz.gov.si/fileadmin/mz.gov.si/pageuploads/javna_razprava_zzDej/ZZDej-1_20.10.2009.doc.

———. 2011. *Nadgradnja zdravstvenega sistema* [Healthcare system upgrade]. Accessed 7 August 2021. http://www.mz.gov.si/fileadmin/mz.gov.si/pageuploads/mz_dokumenti/zakonodaja/Nadgradnja_zdr_sistema_do_2020/HEALTH_SYSTEM_UPGRADE-1.pdf.

———. 2017. *Zakon o spremembah in dopolnitvah zakona o zdravstveni dejavnosti.* Accessed 5 August 2021. http://www.mz.gov.si/si/delovna_podrocja_in_prioritete/zdravstveno_varstvo/zakon_o_spremembah_in_dopolnitvah_zakona_o_zdravstveni_dejavnosti/.

National Assembly. 2007. Voting for Law no. 60/07. Accessed 24 July 2021. https://www.dz-rs.si/wps/portal/Home/seje/izbranoGlasovanje/!ut/p/z1/04_Sj9CPykssy0xPLMnMz0vMAfIjo8zinfyCTD293Q0NLILMDQ0CjT39zHw8DA0D_Q30w8EKvCy9Hb1ACtyNgkwNAl2MnHyDDYwNgoON9KOI0W-AAzgaEKcfj4Io_MYX5IaGhjoqKgIAzEc5Qg!!/dz/d5/L2dBISEvZ0FBIS9nQSEh/?mandat=IV&seja=29.%20Redna&uid=BA201B6502F81BD6C125730200451050.

National Council. 2003. Report on the work of the National Council. Accessed 20 August 2021. http://www.ds-rs.si/sites/default/files/dokumenti/porocilo_ds-2003.doc.

———. 2007. *Državni svet—Bilten*. Accessed 7 August 2021. http://www.ds-rs.si/sites/default/files/dokumenti/biltends_sep07.pdf.

Nova Slovenia. 2017. *Jernej Vrtovec: Opozarjamo na visoke izgube bolnišnic in zahtevamo ukrepanje ministrice* [Jernej Vrtovec: We draw attention to the high losses of hospitals and demand action from the minister]. Accessed 10 August 2021. https://nsi.si/novica/jernej-vrtovec-opozarjamo-na-visoke-izgube-bolnisnic-in-zahtevamo-ukrepanje-ministrice/.

O'Dwyer, Connor. 2014. What accounts for party system stability? Comparing the dimensions of party competition in post-communist Europe. *Europe-Asia Studies* 66 (4): 511–535.

OECD. 2019. *Health expenditure and financing: Health expenditure indicators.* OECD Health Statistics (database). https://doi.org/10.1787/data-00349-en. Accessed 20 September 2019.

Ohranimo. 2006. *Gibanje za ohranitev javnega zdravstva ustanovljeno* [Movement for preservation of public health established]. Accessed 10 August 2021. https://www.ohranimo.si/25/gibanje-za-ohranitev-javnega-zdravstva.html.

Parmelee, Donna E. 1985. Wither the state in Yugoslav health care? *Social Science and Medicine* 21: 719–732.

Parmelee, Donna E. 1989. Yugoslavia: Healthcare under self-managing socialism. In *Success and crisis in national health systems*, ed. M. Field. New York: Routledge.

Parmelee, Donna E., Gail Henderson, and Miron S. Cohen. 1982. Medicine under socialism: Some observations on Yugoslavia and China. *Social Science & Medicine* 16 (15): 1389–1396.

Passaglia, Paolo. 2018. Unicameralism, bicameralism, multicameralism: Evolution and trends in Europe. *Perspectives on Federalism* 10 (2): 1–29.

Popic, Tamara. 2021. Slovenia. In *Health politics in Europe: A handbook*, ed. E.M. Immergut, K.M. Anderson, C. Devitt, and T. Popic. Oxford University Press.

Popic, Tamara and Natalija Perišić. 2021. Former Yugoslavia. In *Health politics in Europe: A handbook*, ed. E.M. Immergut, K.M. Anderson, C. Devitt, and T. Popic, 275–306. Oxford: Oxford University Press.

Prevolnik-Rupel, Valentina. 2018. *ESPN thematic report on inequalities in access to healthcare Slovenia*. Belgium: European Commission.

RTVSLO. 2003. *Keber predstavil belo knjigo* [Keber presented the White Book]. Accessed 7 August 2021. https://www.rtvslo.si/slovenija/keber-predstavil-belo-knjigo/12320.

———. 2006. *Bručan: koncesije niso divja privatizacija* [Bručan: Concessions are not wild privatisation]. Accessed 2 August 2021. https://www.rtvslo.si/slovenija/brucan-koncesije-niso-divja-privatizacija/61178.

———. 2017. *Pobuda za referendum o zakonu o zdravstveni dejavnosti* [Initiative for a referendum on the law on health care activity]. Accessed 15 August 2021. https://www.rtvslo.si/zdravje/pobuda-za-referendum-o-zakonu-o-zdravstveni-dejavnosti-v-dz-ju/433575.

———. 2018. *Ustavno sodišče razveljavilo določbe zakona o zdravstveni dejavnosti* [The Constitutional Court annulled the provisions of the Health Care Activity Act]. Accessed 15 August 2021. https://www.rtvslo.si/zdravje/ustavno-sodisce-razveljavilo-dolocbe-zakona-o-zdravstveni-dejavnosti/475821.

Šarić, Muhamed, and Victor G. Rodwin. 1993. The once and future health system in the former Yugoslavia: Myths and realities. *Journal of Public Health Policy* 14 (2): 220–237.

Slovenian Constitutional Court. 1998. Decision U-I-125/97, 24 June 1998. Accessed 12 August 2021. http://www.us-rs.si/documents/39/35/u-i-125-97-english2.pdf.

———. 2018. Decision U-I-194/17-21, 15 November 2018. Accessed 12 August 2021. https://www.us-rs.si/wp-content/uploads/2020/02/u-i-194-17.pdf.

Stanojević, Miroslav, and Alenka Krašovec. 2011. Slovenia: Social pacts and political exchange. In *Social pacts in Europe: Emergence, evolution, and institutionalization*, ed. S. Avdagic, M. Rhodes, and J. Visser, 232–256. Oxford: Oxford University Press.

Stanovnik, Tine, and Valentina Prevolnik-Rupel. 2014. *ASISP Annual National Report 2014: Pensions, healthcare and long-term care, Slovenia*. Brussels: European Commission.

Stanovnik, Tine, and Eva Turk. 2011. *ASISP Annual National Report 2011: Pensions, health care and long-term care, Slovenia*. Brussels: European Commission.

Štrus, Dušan. 2019. Reshaping the National Council of the Republic of Slovenia. In *Constitutional reform of national legislatures: Bicameralism under pressure*, ed. L. Albert, A. Barragia, and C. Fasone, 230–248. Cheltenham: Edward Elgar Publishing.

Švab, Igor, Irena Vatovec Progar, and Miljana Vegnuti. 2001. Private practice in Slovenia after the health care reform. *The European Journal of Public Health* 11 (4): 407–412.

Svetlik, Ivan. 1989. Od segmentiranih družbenih dejavnosti k pluralnemu sistemu blaginje. In *Prestrukturiranje družbenih dejavnosti*, ed. I. Svetlik, 1–10. Ljubljana: Raziskovalno poročilo ISU.

Toš, Niko. 1991. *Slovensko javno mnenje 1991/1 in 1991/2*. Ljubljana: Fakulteta za družbene vede.

Voljč, Božidar. 1991. Stališča odbora za zdravstvo pri skupščini R Slovenije ob osnutku nove zakonodaje. *Zdravstveni Vestnik* 10: 309.

Zajc, Drago. 2013. Slovenia. In *The handbook of political change in Eastern Europe*, ed. S. Berglund, J. Ekman, K. Deegan-Krause, and T. Knutsen, 339–368. Cheltenham: Edward Elgar Publishing.

CHAPTER 4

The Czech Republic

Introduction

This chapter presents empirical evidence of Czech health policy developments during the post-communist period. Similar to the case of Slovenia, market-oriented reform ideas originated in the socialist period, marking the beginning of a cognitive departure from the paradigm of state-dominated healthcare provision. In contrast to the Slovenian but similar to the Polish policy experience, whilst these ideas were not adopted under socialism, they provided a blueprint for post-communist reforms. However, their translation into policy in the first transitional reforms was a textbook example of market failure in healthcare provision. Subsequent attempts to incorporate market ideas into policy were marked by a series of adjustments and small-scale policy reversals, resulting in a dynamic but instable path of policy development.

To account for this country-specific policy trajectory, the chapter points to the role of legacies, institutions, and politics (see Chap. 2). It explains that the post-communist reformers lacked policy experience other than that associated with the state-dominated healthcare system. They opted for radical market reforms, but these were plagued by implementation failures and needed adjustment. Further attempts to introduce market elements in Czech healthcare were shaped by polarised, yet moderate political conflict and medium strong institutional constraints. The party relations in the healthcare arena showed both divisions and pragmatic

T. Popic, *Health Reforms in Post-Communist Eastern Europe*,
https://doi.org/10.1007/978-3-031-15497-3_4

compromises, making the Czech case different from the Polish one, where these divisions were stronger (see Chap. 5), and from Slovenia, where they were weak (Chap. 3). This party dynamic was combined with institutional configurations that concentrated policymaking within Parliament, whilst party conflicts were resolved by the Czech Constitutional Court. This contributed to an unstable policy path that was less protracted than Poland's pattern of reversals, but more turbulent than Slovenia's pattern of the survival of market reforms despite challenges.

The chapter proceeds as follows. It first provides an overview of the Czech healthcare system under socialism, presenting the main policy debates in this period and accounting for the emergence of market-oriented policy ideas. The chapter then discusses four main episodes of market-oriented reforms during the three post-communist decades: introduction of managed competition, privatisation of primary care, establishment of user fees for medical services, and hospital privatisation. The conclusion summarises the main findings, links these findings with the core argument of the book, and compares the Czech case to the Polish and Slovenian cases of health policy learning in post-communism.

Czech Healthcare Under Socialism

The initial phase of Czech health policy development under socialism implied a gradual but systemic adaptation of the Soviet 'Semashko model' of state-dominated healthcare provision.[1] While close adherence to the Soviet model contributed to impressive post-war improvements in population health outcomes, the improvements were short-lived, and the healthcare system began to show anomalies, such as shortages and corruption. The growing crisis of the health sector stimulated criticism and led to the emergence of market-oriented policy ideas, generating the first cracks in the socialist paradigm. The crisis continued to grow throughout the 1980s, leading to further discussion on possible solutions to policy problems. There was little political will to change, so the emerging market ideas did not translate into actual polices. Nevertheless, they provided a basis for reform in post-communism.

[1] Nikolai Semashko was the founder of the healthcare system in the Soviet Union, serving as the People's Commissar of Public Health from 1918 to 1930.

Introduction of the Socialist Policy Paradigm

Throughout the early post-war period, the Czech health system was gradually re-modelled to fit the Soviet model of healthcare based on planned, centralised, and state-dominated provision of medical services.[2] The first post-war changes occurred shortly after the end of the German occupation, when in 1945, the provisional Czechoslovak government nationalised existing private health insurance funds.[3] The next move towards the establishment of the Soviet-style healthcare model were taken after the Communist Party of Czechoslovakia seized power in the 1946 elections and the 1948 coup d'état sealed the communist rule of the country. The 1948 Law on National Insurance centralised healthcare financing by abolishing the existing model of multiple health insurance funds and established one central fund, the Central National Insurance Fund (Alexa et al. 2015: 18). A further step towards the state-dominated model took place in 1951 with the Law on Budget, which abolished the Central National Insurance Fund and incorporated healthcare financing into the state budget, switching from contributions to general revenues as the main source of system financing (see also Bryndová et al. 2019).

Integration of healthcare financing into the state budget gave the post-war healthcare system a distinctively statist, hierarchical, and rigid form. Financing through taxes meant the State Planning Commission was responsible for the management of healthcare financing on the basis of a normative Five-Year Plan. Under this Plan, the Ministry of Finance developed an annual state budget for healthcare and through the Ministry of the Interior, it allocated funds to local authorities—Regional and District National Committees—which then distributed the relevant funds to the Regional and District Institutes of National Health under their jurisdiction. Centralisation and state control were ensured, as the directors of these institutes were appointed by the heads of the above-mentioned national committees, after receiving approval from the Communist Party (Jaroš and Kalina 1998).

The post-war changes in healthcare provision reflected a close adherence to the Soviet model as well. As healthcare facilities were nationalised, healthcare professionals became state employees, and the Ministry began

[2] Czech Republic was part of the Czechoslovak Republic, in 1960 renamed the federal Czechoslovak Socialist Republic, from 1948 to 1990.

[3] During the inter-war period, healthcare in the First Czechoslovak Republic was provided through private, occupation-based health insurance funds (Inglot 2008: 68).

to control the professional aspects of healthcare, such as regulation of salaries of healthcare professionals and allocation of drugs and medical supplies to healthcare facilities.[4] A distinctive Czechoslovak element in the organisation of healthcare provision was that the nationalisation of healthcare facilities was followed by their administrative incorporation into a new type of institution—Institutes of National Health. As facilities were incorporated into the Regional and District Institutes of National Health, these institutes were responsible at the district and regional levels, respectively, whilst the Ministry of Health took administrative responsibility at the national level (Marrée and Groenewegen 1997: 53). Healthcare services at the local level were organised through community health centres and delivered according to strictly defined territorial rules. Another Soviet feature was the strong focus on occupational medicine—enterprise physicians and facilities—with the goal to deliver preventive and curative care for industrial workers. Universal coverage meant health services were free, with a few exceptions for services deemed to be 'not indispensable' such as, for example, implantation of dental gold (Käser 1976; Jaroš and Kalina 1998).

The post-war remake of the Czechoslovak health system led to significant improvements, most visible in terms of population coverage, infrastructure, manpower, and financing. The extension of coverage, for example, meant 93 per cent of the Czechoslovak population had healthcare coverage by 1950 (Käser 1976).[5] The country adopted another Soviet-style element of health policy: a focus on public health and hygiene (Field 1991). Together, these elements led to impressive achievements in population health. From 1938 to 1965, Czechoslovak male life expectancy increased from 55 to 68 years and infant mortality rates dropped dramatically from 113 to 25 deaths in first year of life per 1000 live births, one of the largest declines in infant mortality globally (Weinerman 1969: 44).

[4] Private medical practice was officially forbidden, but the Minister of Health could give a license for private practice to 'outstanding' specialists, such as retired doctors and dental surgeons. These private doctors offered services to those not covered by the public system—until 1966 the self-employed and agricultural workers—and those able to pay for private services (see Popic 2021).

[5] This was an impressive achievement, as in 1938, only 22 per cent of the population was covered (Korbel 1997: 78, author's calculation).

These successes of the post-war health policy were crowned by the introduction of the 1966 Law on Health of the Population.[6] This law established the legal base for universal healthcare provision; it stipulated healthcare was a basic right guaranteed by the Constitution and, as such, was to be provided by the state, free of charge, to all citizens (Käser 1976).[7] Implementation of this law led to expansion of coverage to the previously excluded categories of self-employed and agricultural workers, making the post-war healthcare system a fully universal one. The universal coverage was coupled with what was described at the time as a 'remarkably uniform and stable' pattern of healthcare organisation, which 'succeeded in bringing to the entire population extensive range of health benefits without relying on supplementary individual payments or private professional practice' (Weinerman 1969: 77–79).

The Socialist Healthcare Crisis

Paradoxically, the strengths of the socialist healthcare system soon became the main source of its problems. The first issues in healthcare provision emerged in the late 1960s and included a lack of material resources and inflexibility in the adaptation of national policies to local needs (Weinerman 1969). These issues became even more visible during the 1970s, and the system's incapacity to respond to the population's health needs was soon reflected in health outcomes, as indicators such as life expectancy stagnated, and mortality indicators signalled worsening population health (Jaroš and Kalina 1998). By the 1980s, the situation in the sector was alarming, with standardised mortality rates reaching close to 1300 deaths per 100,000 inhabitants, two times higher than the mortality rates in Western Europe (Jaroš and Kalina 1998: 4; see also Gibbons 1993). The decline in population health was coupled with chronic shortages of medical services and medicines, and this, in turn, led to corruption, with patients making under-the-table payments in return for treatment (Raffel and Raffel 1992; Svobodný et al. 2004). The contrast between the communist model of universally provided, free healthcare and the reality of deteriorating population health and a healthcare system plagued by shortages and corruption became increasingly obvious.

[6] *Zákon o péči o zdraví lidu*, Law No. 20/1966.
[7] Law 20/1966, Article V.

Emergence of Market Ideas

The first voices mentioning the cracks in the Soviet healthcare policy paradigm were heard in the 1980s. Charter 77 (*Charta 77*) was the only anti-regime dissident group active in communist Czechoslovakia from the late 1970s.[8] In 1984, the Charter published a letter addressed to the Czech National Council and the Ministry of Health, accompanied by a 14-page document, 'Health is Part of the Right to Life', prepared by an anonymous group belonging to the organisation (Charter 77 1984). The letter emphasised the need for a discussion of the situation in the healthcare sector, expressing the prevailing feelings of the population as follows: 'What happened to our health system? It used to be our pride!' (Charter 77 1984: iv).

The accompanying document analysed the health sector's problems and suggested solutions. Referring to the sector's developments during the post-war period and to the 1966 law, the analysis underlined the core principles of the socialist health system according to which as health is part of the right to life, the state has a duty to guarantee provision of health services adequate to meet this right. The document then contrasted the state's responsibility with the current state of affairs in the Czech health sector, describing it as progressively deteriorating due to insufficient financing, misallocation of resources, shortage of medicines, lack of modern medical equipment, and a growing black market of healthcare goods and services. Pointing to these as obstacles in the system's ability to deliver care, it called for the identification of the real causes of the sector's shortcomings (Charter 77 1984). The authors did not mince words:

> We have so consistently implemented a system whose poor functioning has its own causes. At the beginning, it could seem like progress and it could work satisfactorily. Over the years, however, the consequences of those built-in systemic disorders have been catastrophically accumulating, bureaucratic nonsense has become more acute, and the whole crisis is being accelerated by new scientific knowledge, the increasing technical demands of modern medicine and the expanding range of new therapies and options. It turns out that the system, on the one hand, restricts freedom and binds the initiative of the individual, and on the other hand, it does not satisfy either the general public or the abstract interest of society. (Charter 77 1984: xvi)

[8] This movement was founded in 1977 by a group of Czechoslovak intellectuals including, among others, the future President of the post-communist Czech Republic, Václav Havel.

The document further argued the problems of the health sector were not just 'negative phenomena', as labelled by the authorities, but rather 'a symptom of a dysfunctional system'. The reasons for this dysfunctionality, it said, lay in the core principles of the socialist health policy, its hierarchical character, and the state's monopoly on health system organisation. Concluding its analysis, it said the crisis of the health sector was simply an expression of a much wider crisis of the socialist establishment, which could be resolved only through reforms on a broader societal level (Charter 77 1984: xvi).

The criticisms expressed in Charter 77's document were clearly an opposition group's way of challenging the main underpinnings of the socialist system, but they also expressed wider public concerns about the health sector. The document was effective, as one year after its publication, Czech Minister of Health[9] Jaroslav Prokopec commissioned a report to analyse the healthcare sector's main problems and suggest possible solutions. The report was commissioned to a group of experts from the Institute of Social Medicine and Healthcare Organisation, a state organisation which conducted regular analyses of the sector. Once published, echoing the Charter's document, the report pointed to low and unsatisfactory system performance, linking it to a more general worsening of the population's health status and accompanying problems, such as inequalities in healthcare financing and provision across the regions. In contrast to the Charter's analysis, however, this report remained faithful to the socialist policy paradigm. Rather than proposing a systemic reform, it simply suggested that the government should find ways to ensure additional financing for the health sector.[10]

According to one of the authors of the report, this was just the official version of the experts' view. The experts knew the health system needed a more systemic change, but they also knew that recommending any type of systemic change would be considered 'heresy', and they might lose their jobs. Moreover, the policy experts did not think any political change involving a departure from the socialist policy model was even possible.[11] In other words, the experts were aware that the authorities needed suggestions that would stay within the limits of the existing policy paradigm, and

[9] Czechoslovakia was federalised in 1968, and each federal state had its own Ministry of Health.

[10] Interview No. 9.

[11] Interview No. 9.

proposing departures from this paradigm would be too risky and unlikely to materialise.

Continued adherence to the existing policy paradigm marked the policy debates of the late 1980s. As healthcare continued to deteriorate, healthcare issues moved to the top of the government agenda. In November 1988, the Czech National Council published a resolution admitting that the worsening of public health was a source of justified public criticism (Czech National Council 1988). At subsequent meetings of the Council, healthcare was one of the burning issues of debate. At the Council's meeting in December 1988, Chairman of the Health and Social Committee Josef Domas blamed the worsening of population health on factors outside the healthcare system, such as lifestyle and eating habits. He further argued that the main cause of the healthcare problem was the 'suboptimal dualism' of the existing system in which the Ministry of Health had overall responsibility for healthcare, but the networks of healthcare facilities were administered by regional and district health authorities. Domas proposed stricter centralisation, giving more power to the Ministry of Health and less to the healthcare facilities networks, but he was pessimistic about the overall prospects of the sector, given the meagre increase in the healthcare budget planned for 1989 (Domas 1988).

The discussions of the socialist healthcare policy in the 1980s demonstrated an awareness of a real crisis in the health sector among the wider public, medical professionals, experts, and even the political elites. In other words, there was a general recognition of the anomalies in the existing policy paradigm. These discussions generated proposals that argued for even stronger centralisation, however, and the government solutions were clearly confined within the existing paradigm of centralised, hierarchical, and bureaucratic healthcare provision. This situation was best summarised by one of the experts as follows:

> During the 1980s, there were no considerable changes even though there was large amount of deep research conducted about the situation in the healthcare sector. None of the research results however ended on the table of the decision makers, because the party structure was too frightened to change things.[12]

[12] Interview No. 8.

The months preceding the regime change in 1989 hinted at possible departures from the existing healthcare model. In an interview in June 1989, Minister of Health Prokopec admitted that the financial crisis of the health sector was the worst crisis experienced during his 19-year mandate (ČTK 1989a). In a subsequent interview, he proposed concrete solutions. For example, additional funding for the sector could be generated by introducing two types of patient co-payments: general patient co-payments for non-essential services and drugs, such as cosmetic surgery and vitamins, and special co-payments for essential health services of population groups with risky health behaviour, such as smokers and heavy drinkers (ČTK 1989b). The Minister's proposals clearly contrasted with the socialist paradigm and suggested the model of universal, publicly provided healthcare was increasingly seen as untenable even by the socialist authorities. Moreover, these proposals emerged just a few months before the regime-breaking events of 1989, thus suggesting the socialist paradigm was imploding. This implosion became even more vigorous in the aftermath of the Velvet Revolution.

Institutional and Political Contexts of Post-Communist Health Reform

As radical reforms were deemed politically unfavourable, the health sector did not change under socialism, and this policy stagnation contributed to the troubled nature of the first post-communist reforms. The Czech transitional reformers enthusiastically opted for radical solutions, but they lacked experience. Their reforms generated text-book examples of market failure and threw the health system into crisis. Fortunately, they were able to regulate the market forces and put the new system on its feet relatively quickly. The troubled beginning was followed by a bumpy but nevertheless continuous trajectory of reform aimed at integrating elements of privatisation and competition into a new insurance-based system of healthcare provision.

As argued in this book, the post-communist reform trajectory of Slovakia, Czech Republic, and Poland is best understood as learning which involves the adaptation of reform ideas, shaped by the institutional and political setup of the policymaking process. The 1992 Czech Constitution established the country as an independent state and specified medium strong institutional veto configurations featuring bicameralism, weak presidential powers, and a judiciary vested with veto powers through Constitutional Court. This institutional setting, in combination with political parties' division over policy issues but readiness for pragmatic compromises, deeply affected the dynamics of policy learning in the Czech case. The parliament's Lower House, the Chamber of Deputies, became the key policymaking arena, whilst party conflicts were resolved by the Constitutional Court. The main result of this setup was an instable pattern of policy learning.

Institutions: Medium Strong Veto Points Configurations

The post-communist institutional design was introduced soon after the breakup of the Federal state. The 1992 Constitution instituted a bicameral parliamentary system comprised of the Lower House, the Chamber of Deputies (*Poslanecká sněmovna*), and the Upper House, the Senate (*Senát*).[13] It granted the Chamber the right to prepare and pass legislation with the absolute majority of votes, and the Senate the right of veto over the Chamber's decisions, but the Senate's veto could be overturned by an absolute majority of votes in the Chamber. Similarly, the Constitution vested the President as the head of State with veto powers over the Chamber's decisions, but President's veto depended on the support of the majority of votes in the Chamber. The Czech Constitutional Court was granted the right to veto laws it judged incompatible with the Constitution. Lastly, the Constitution granted the electorate the possibility to reject government's decisions through a public referendum (Constitution of the Czech Republic 1992).

The constitutional rules which gave the Senate and the President only weak conditional veto powers over the Chamber of Deputies' decisions implied that the policymaking developed primarily within the government and the Chamber as Parliament's Lower House. This institutional setup, in combination with the electoral laws establishing a proportional electoral system, provided for a strong form of party government (Kopecký 2007: 143). In health policy, this meant the Chamber was the key decision-making arena; it also meant the political composition and strength of the government relative to the opposition were key factors shaping the

[13] The Senate was introduced in a 1993 amendment to the Constitution (Czech Constitution 1993).

direction of Czech health policy throughout the post-communist period (see Popic 2021).

The only institution able to control the Chamber's health policy decisions was the Czech Constitutional Court. As this chapter goes on to show, the role of the Constitutional Court was significant in two different policy episodes. One involved the recurring issue of user fees, patients' payments for medical services. Initially, the Court judged these payments were unconstitutional because they conflicted with the constitutional right to free healthcare (Czech Constitutional Court 1995), but in a subsequent dispute, it changed its position, arguing the user fees introduced in the 2007 Law on Public Budget Stabilisation were not in conflict with the Constitution (Czech Constitutional Court 2008). In 2013, the Court opposed an increase in user fees for hospital services, arguing this policy move threatened access to healthcare for vulnerable groups (Czech Constitutional Court 2013). The Court also played a significant role in the context of hospital transformation, judging attempts to block commercialisation of public hospitals were unconstitutional, because they interfered with constitutional property rights and rights of self-governance of the regions (Czech Constitutional Court 2008).

The veto of the Czech President was constitutionally weaker but still came into play in the policymaking process. For example, President Václav Klaus vetoed the 2003 law blocking hospital transformation, even though his vetoe was subsequently overturned in the Chamber of Deputies. This confirmed the key role of party politics and the role of the Chamber as the main decision-making arena. In a comparative perspective, this stands in stark contrast to Poland where, as shown in the next chapter (see Chap. 5), the President's veto powers were constitutionally stronger and hence played a decisive role in shaping health policy.

Party Politics: Moderate Party Divide on Health Policy

Czechoslovak communist leadership collapsed unexpectedly, capitulating after the peaceful mass protests on the streets of Prague in the so-called Velvet Revolution in November 1989 (Stark and Bruszt 1998: 18). This sudden capitulation came as a surprise to Civic Forum (*Občanské fórum—OF*), an opposition group led by Václav Havel. It had organised anti-regime demonstrations paving the way to the Velvet Revolution, and it took part in the subsequent Round Table Talks with the regime. The outcome of the Talks was momentous, as negotiators agreed on the formation of a government coalition and the replacement of a share of communist deputies in both the Federal Assembly and the Czech National Council by the members of the opposition (Calda 1996).[14] The extrication from socialism was followed by another major political event marking the beginning of the post-communist period: the peaceful breakup of the federal state on 25 November 1992. The peaceful dissolution of the federal state and the adoption of a new Constitution on 16 December 1992 contributed to a relatively smooth political transition.

The 1995 electoral law established a moderate system of proportional representation that tempered political party fragmentation by creating strong party discipline and lower incentives to form smaller parties (Keefer and Shirley 2001). This electoral system was structured to favour larger parties and produced a relatively stable pattern of political competition. As a result, the Czech post-communist party system consolidated quickly and remained fairly stable during the first two post-communist decades (Casal Bértoa 2011). Similar to Slovenia (Chap. 3), the main party conflict was between communists and non-communists. The first post-communist elections, held in 1990, were considered more a public plebiscite on communist rule than an open competition between different parties (Bugajski 2002: 233). The elections resulted in a sweeping victory of the various anti-communist forces under the Civic Forum, suggesting the conflict would be short-lived (see Mansfeldová 2013).

The clear dominance of the anti-communists in the first post-communist government meant the elites were given a green light for large-scale transitional restructuring. This, in turn, triggered a shift from the communist versus non-communist conflict to one focused on more concrete social and economic issues. The 1992 election signalled the concrete move of political competition towards the socio-economic dimension, as the various political parties had clearly positioned themselves on a traditional left-right axis. The main result of this political dynamic was an early crystallisation of party positions on socio-economic issues, with parties competing on positions clustered around questions of social security, redistribution of resources, and the role of the state (Kopecký 2007: 120).

In those early years, several new political parties emerged from the fragmented anti-communist block, whilst some of the country's old political forces remained and were revived. The strongest right-wing partisan

[14] The 1990 Czech elections were fully free, in contrast to the 1991 Polish elections where only part of the Sejm's seats were open for the competition (see Chap. 5).

formation deriving from the anti-communist block was the liberal-conservative Civic Democratic Party (*Občanská demokratická strana—ODS*), led by Václav Klaus, the first post-communist Federal Minister of Finance. The ODS profile was shaped by Klaus, whose radical policies of the early 1990s were credited for the country's speedy economic liberalisation and privatisation. The party was committed to reducing the role of the state in the economy, and it strongly supported privatisation and the right of individual (Bugajski 2002: 245). Thanks to the power of Klaus' leadership and the party's key role in the transition, the ODS soon eliminated its like-minded political rivals (e.g., Civic Democratic Alliance, *Občanská demokratická alliance—ODA*) and became the leading political force on the right side of the political spectrum.

On the left, the Czech Social Democratic Party (*Česká strana sociálně demokratická—ČSSD*) evolved into the strongest political actor and a weighty rival to the ODS (Mansfeldová 2013: 225). Unlike other social democratic parties in the former Eastern Bloc, the ČSSD did not emerge from the former communist party; in fact, its historical origins dated back to the First Czechoslovak Republic.[15] Having roots in the pre-communist social democratic tradition implied the party had organisational and ideological continuity, and this contributed to the ČSSD's ability to identify itself as a genuinely social democratic party and to promote 'Western style', 'Third Way' policies. In other words, it took a social-market approach which relied on a balanced combination of solidarity and individual responsibility and a more statist approach marked by, for example, generous welfare funding (Cabada 2010).

ČSSD's efforts to be recognised as a genuinely social democratic party significantly contributed to the party's electoral success, making it the dominant party on the left of the ideological spectrum (Kopeček and Pšeja 2008). This ideological profile meant the ČSSD's conflict with the ODS, and thus the overall conflict dominating the inter-party competition, revolved around the issue of the role of the state versus market liberalism, a conflict which overlapped with the left-right division of the political spectrum (Kitschelt et al. 1999; Mansfeldová 2013). The ČSSD had to share the left side of the political spectrum with the old communists, the

[15] The ČSSD was founded in 1878 as the Czechoslovak Social Democratic Party within the Austrian Social Democratic Party. The party was dissolved in 1938, restored in 1945, forcibly merged with the Communist Party of Czechoslovakia in 1948, and then resumed its activities on 19 November 1989 (Bugajski 2002: 241).

communist successor party, the Communist Party of Bohemia and Moravia (*Komunistická strana Čech a Moravy—KSČM*), but it did not want to be identified with the communists. Therefore, it rejected coalitions with KSČM even when the latter was the only other leftist party with parliamentary representation. This unwillingness to cooperate with the communists in order to preserve the party's social democratic identity severely constrained the ČSSD's coalition potential.[16]

More generally, the development of the socio-economic dimension as the main axis of party competition quite soon in the transition had a significant impact on health politics. The main party conflict over health policy was between the two strongest political rivals, the ODS and the ČSSD. The conflict developed in the early 1990s and was present throughout the three post-communist decades. The source of the conflict was, simply stated, ideological. As noted above, the parties' ideological profiles overlapped with the traditional left-right division; not surprisingly, then, the ČSSD's conflict with the ODS revolved around the issue of the role of the state versus market liberalism. The ODS quickly became the main party advocating market reforms in the healthcare sector, whilst the ČSSD served as the ODS's major political counter-force, defending a vision of a more public, solidaristic, and universal healthcare system. This two-party conflict over health policy remained more or less stable, as both parties continued to win almost equivalent share of votes—ranging from 25 to 35 per cent. As time passed, the health policy debate continued to be dominated by the ODS and the ČSSD, suggesting the parties' ownership of health issues remained relatively unchanged despite the arrival of new parties and the re-alignment of Czech party politics during the third post-communist decade.[17]

Yet, the stability of party competition and the ČSSD's insistence on its social democratic identity also contributed to the moderation of the parties' divide over health policy. The stability of the party system meant the party competition for most of the post-communist period was characterised by the continual parliamentary presence of four parties with standard

[16] Non-cooperation with the communists was formally established in the ČSSD's 1995 Bohumín resolution (Kopeček and Pšeja 2008).

[17] From 1992 to 2019, the only two Ministers of Health not belonging to either ODS or ČSSD were Leoš Heger, from the TOP09 party (Tradition, Responsibility, Prosperity; *Tradice Odpovědnost Prosperita*) who was Minister of Health from 2010 to 2013, and Adam Vojtěch, from ANO 2011 (Action of Dissatisfied Citizens; *Akce nespokojených občanů*), Minister of Health from 2017 to 2020.

political profiles—the two leading parties, the ODS and the ČSSD, were joined by the Christian democratic KDU-ČSL (a coalition of Christian and Democratic Union and the Czechoslovak People's Party) and the communist KSČM (Hanley 2012). Given its ideological affiliations, the ODS usually formed governing coalitions with the Christian Democrats, KDU-ČSL, and this linkage made it temper its policy positions. In a similar manner, because of its social democratic identity, the ČSSD rejected cooperation with the KSČM[18] and made governing coalitions with the KDU-ČSL and, during the third post-communist decade, with a new liberal party, Action of Dissatisfied Citizens (*Akce nespokojených občanů—ANO 2011*), all of which made it move towards the centre (see Kopecký 2007). When there was lack of coalition potential, or if conflict emerged in a coalition, the ODS and the ČSSD would even rely on one another. The survival of the 1996–1997 ODS government, for example, depended on the support of the ČSSD, who struck an informal unwritten agreement to support the government. Similarly, the ODS had a formal written agreement to support the 1998–2002 ČSSD government. Both cross-party agreements, especially the 1996–1997 agreement, were crucial for health policy, as they tempered the ODS' market zeal and enabled a shift from a managed competition model to a more regulated system of health-care provision.

The ODS-ČSSD dominance of the health policy debate meant the parties had a monopoly on the policymaking process and thus could apply exclusionary tactics in response to the demands of professional interests (see Kopecký 2007). These tactics aimed at downplaying or eliminating the role of the unions and professional associations in policymaking and were evident, for example, in the weak role of the tripartite bodies in the early health reforms. The use of exclusionary tactics was facilitated by interest fragmentation, as the privatisation of primary care contributed to professional divisions between doctors working in the public and private sectors. The consequence was that the voices of health professionals were not heard in the formal policymaking process. As the chapter goes on to show, doctors were unsuccessful in their attempts to steer health policy direction. They were unable to prevent abolition of the fee-for-service system, an extremely lucrative reimbursement method introduced in the early 1990s. Nor could they prevent the introduction of user fees in the

[18] The KSČM was the only Czech party systematically excluded from every government coalition, gaining the status of political 'pariah' (Casal Bértoa 2014: 15).

2000s, a measure they opposed, as they feared it would interfere with their relationship with patients. Unheard in formal venues, the health professionals expressed their views of health reform in strikes and protests to put pressure on the government. These protests usually focused on issues of pay or working conditions and rarely dealt with more systemic reforms which, as shown in this chapter, were essentially shaped by the parties' vision of health policy and institutional constraints.

In the Czech case, the conflict between the main political forces was much more pronounced than in the Slovenian case (see Chap. 3), but the Polish party divide was much stronger, putting Czech Republic somewhere in the middle. In contrast to the Polish communist successor party SLD (see Chap. 5), the ČSSD had continuous ownership of health policy issues but never advocated a return to a state-dominated, centralised healthcare system. Rather, its role in health policy focused on counterbalancing the strong pro-market stance of the ODS, but because of its 'Third Way' approach, it also showed readiness to accept some market elements, such as certain types of user fees and consumer-oriented policies of patient rights. For its part, the ODS contributed to the moderation of the party divide by being willing to scale down its pro-market advocacy in the face of implementation failures and lack of political support. The combination of this moderate partisan divide and a medium strong institutional veto setup prevented systemic reversals, but contributed to instable transformation in the healthcare system.

Key Episodes in Post-Communist Healthcare Reform

Initial Post-Communist Reform Debates

The first initiatives for large-scale transformation of the health system emerged in the immediate aftermath of the November 1989 Velvet Revolution. An organisation actively involved in the reform initiative was part of the Civic Forum, called the Civic Forum of Health Professionals (*Občanské fórum zdravotníků—OFZ*). The Prague branch of OFZ published a document entitled 'Theses on the Healthcare Programme' in January 1990.[19] Building on the independent experts' reports from the 1980s discussed earlier in the chapter, this document pointed to a crisis in

[19] *Teze k programu zdraví. Praha, Programová skupina Občanského fóra zdravotníků, Svazyčeských lékařů a Zväzu slovenských lekárov. Zdravotnické noviny* 29(4), 26 January 1990.

the health sector and stressed the need for its solution, emphasising the need for public debate on measures to find a way out of the crisis. The measures it proposed included, among others, abolition of the state monopoly, de-bureaucratisation, and the shift to a new form of health system organisation based on insurance.[20]

Another organisation that became actively involved in developing proposals for health reform was the Institute of Social Medicine and Organisation of Health Care, a state institution which in the late 1980s published reports commissioned by the Ministry of Health. A group of expert from this Institute, composed of sociologists and economists, became advisors to Pavel Klener, the first post-communist Minister of Health in the temporary cabinet of Peter Pithart. In May 1990, this expert group published ‘A Proposal for Reforming Healthcare’. It was more concrete than the OFZ document as it advocated a shift to a system of social health insurance based on multiple insurance funds and suggested both mandatory and voluntary health insurance as options for healthcare coverage (Potůček 1999: 115). Health insurance contributions would be subtracted from workers’ salaries; other suggested sources of financing included state and local budgets and patient co-payments.

The document proposed two options for healthcare delivery reform, with an implementation timeline of four to five years. Both options entailed the dissolution of the existing Regional and District Institutes for National Health and a bottom-up formation of a new organisational structure of healthcare delivery. In the first option, healthcare facilities would become independent public institutions; they would organise themselves into Associations of Health Care Facilities to optimise healthcare provision within a given area. The existing health authorities would be replaced by Health Councils who would develop the overall health policy for a given area, approve the budgets of the Associations, and nominate candidates for administration. Health Councils would be made up of local councillors, health professionals, and representatives of health organisations. In the second option, municipalities and local communities would assume the ownership and administration of healthcare facilities in their territory. Finally, the document recommended devolving oversight of the medical profession from the state to an autonomous chamber of physicians (Ministry of Health 1990a).

[20] Interview No. 8.

In the June 1990 elections, the first multiparty elections in post-communist Czechoslovakia, the Civic Forum posted a stunning victory, with almost 50 per cent of the total vote, thus confirming the victory of the anti-communists. The large mandate of the Civic Forum—127 seats in the Czech National Council—gave the new government, formed again under Pithart, a crucial boost to continue its reform efforts. Pithart's government appointed Martin Bojar, one of the key activists of the Velvet Revolution and one of the leaders of the OFZ, as the first post-communist Minister of Health. Bojar's Ministry enjoyed a high degree of autonomy, as shortly after the elections, the former Ministry of Health and Social Affairs was divided into two institutions—the Ministry of Health and the Ministry of Labour and Social Affairs (Jaroš et al. 2005). Whilst Bojar's Ministerial position signalled that the departure from the socialist system of healthcare was high on the winning party's agenda, the appointment of Kamil Kalina as Deputy Health Minister and Director of the Health Policy Department was more crucial in shaping the actual direction of healthcare reforms. Kalina was a part of the fraction of the Civic Forum which gathered its more right-wing members around Václav Klaus, the Forum's Chairman and the federal Minister of Finance in the new Czechoslovak government. Kalina quickly emerged as the leader of the Ministry's reform team, advocating a more radical and liberal approach to health reforms.[21]

This approach was immediately apparent in a reform document Kalina's team published in October 1990, 'Proposal for a New Health Care System' (Ministry of Health 1990b). Clearly building on the proposal prepared by Klener's expert team from the Institute of Social Medicine, the document recommended the introduction of health insurance system, but unlike the Institute's proposal, it envisaged a radical departure from the state-dominated model. More specifically, it proposed the introduction of an insurance system composed of multiple funds, some of which would be public, whilst others, in order to spur competition, would be private. The plan also envisaged competition among healthcare providers according to the 'money follows the patient' principle; to this end, it proposed setting up a competitive, fee-for-service (FFS) reimbursement method. Much like the previous proposal, in healthcare delivery, the plan included the dissolution of the Regional and District Institutes for National Health and a bottom-up formation of a new local government structure for healthcare facilities. It did not make specific provisions for ownership arrangements,

[21] Interview No. 8.

stating that most healthcare facilities would retain their public ownership, but also outlining the possibility of the transfer of facilities to local authorities, who would then be free to decide whether to privatise them or not.[22]

Almost simultaneously, a competitive proposal emerged. This proposal was prepared by the same group of experts from the Institute for Social Medicine and Healthcare Organisation who prepared the May 1990 proposal. This proposal was much less in favour of competition and suggested the new system should feature territorially based insurance funds and remunerate health services through a mix based on salaries, capitation fees, and fee-for-service.

The more liberal and market-oriented proposal of the Ministerial team was more successful because it was favoured by Finance Minister Klaus (Jaroš et al. 2005). Klaus held a position in the federal government, and as the newly elected Chairman of the Civic Forum, he was one of its most influential members. Not surprisingly given his position of power, he emerged as the leader of the Czech neo-liberal transition to capitalism. His support for the plan offered by Kalina's team significantly contributed to its success, so that just two months after its publication, in December 1990, the Ministry team's proposal was accepted as the government's official programme for healthcare reform.

The vying proposals were evidence of a lively policy debate among Czech experts, but the international expert community was trying to offer reform advice as well. The World Bank, for example, was very interested in giving a hand to Czech policymakers. The Bank's experts visited the country in January 1991 and met with local healthcare experts and the Minister of Health. The result of this visit was published in a report outlining the healthcare sector reform priorities and suggesting concrete reforms (World Bank 1991).

As the Bank saw it, the most urgent priority was to survive the period of economic instability likely to accompany the transition to a market economy. Suggesting a gradual approach to health reforms, the Bank's report distinguished between short- and medium-term measures. Short-term measures, labelled top priority and, as such, to be introduced immediately to prevent the collapse of the health sector, focused on policies of cost-containment to improve efficiency and eliminate waste (World Bank 1991). One of the recommended cost-containment measures was the introduction of different types of co-payment, the most important of

[22] Interview No. 8.

which would be co-payment for medicine. The Bank's experts considered the price of medicine was vulnerable to price liberalisation, the deregulation of pharmaceutical industry, inflation, and currency devaluation. They saw uncontrolled increases of expenditure on medicine as presenting a serious threat to the sector's stability and insisted on control as the only way of preventing large deficits. The idea was that these short-term measures would pave the way to medium-term reforms. These latter reforms included privatisation of healthcare delivery, seen as a way of abolishing corruption. In healthcare financing, medium-term reforms included the gradual reduction of funding from general revenues and a shift to funding from compulsory health insurance contributions and other sources (World Bank 1991).

The Bank's experts took a much more cautious approach to the introduction of health insurance than the country's experts. The Bank saw health insurance as a way of making the health sector more autonomous and less vulnerable to political machinations, but its experts warned against false illusions that could be created by what they called the 'magic of insurance', stressing that a shift to a social insurance model would not make equity and efficiency easier to achieve (World Bank 1991). In fact, they advocated a measured approach to the introduction of competitive reimbursement mechanisms, such as fee-for-service and capitation. These mechanisms, the experts argued, might provide incentives to stimulate performance, but their actual impact on efficiency, expenditure, and quality of care was unknown. In addition, they ran the risk of creating perverse incentives. They also warned about the downside of private insurance, stressing that, unless heavily regulated, private insurance might encourage 'cream skimming' of low-risk populations, leaving the public sector with the heaviest burden in the provision of care (World Bank 1991). The Bank's formulation of a cautious approach to the introduction of a competitive insurance system was succinct: 'If left unregulated, health insurance has considerable potential for leading to a major health expenditure escalation, which is not desirable during the period of economic stabilisation' (World Bank 1991: 46).

Concluding its analysis of the health sector, the Bank report argued that reforms would not be possible without both foreign expertise and capital, suggesting the funding of the reform process could be supported by international institutions, such as the World Bank or the World Health Organisation (World Bank 1991). In fact, shortly after the experts' visit, the World Bank offered a loan for health reform in exchange for oversight of the reform process. However, the offer was rejected, as the Bank's proposals were not received favourably in domestic policy circles.

This hostile attitude to foreign advice reflected the more general hostility of the government's officials to recommendations from international organisations. Stating its reason for rejecting the World Bank's offer of a loan, the government emphasised its firm belief that prudent financial policy should be focused on avoiding loans and approaching debts cautiously. It mistrusted views from abroad and consequently did not accept international expert intervention in national policy.[23] This general rejection of foreign advice is perhaps best summarised in Václav Klaus's famous comment that he was 'not ready to pay hard money for soft advice' (Klaus 2018). The effect of this, as this chapter shows next, was that Czech reformers ignored most, if not all, recommendations for health policy reform given by the World Bank's experts. What is more, their subsequent policy choices generated text-book examples of market failure—the very thing the Bank's report specifically warned against.

Introduction of Social Health Insurance and Managed Competition

Despite clear warnings from international experts, the core of the government's approach was a strongly market-oriented idea according to which minimum market regulation would lead to an optimal health system (see Jaroš and Kalina 1998: 4). Following the acceptance of the Ministry's proposal as an official government programme for reform, Kalina's team started working on a set of bills. The drafting of the new reform plans took place in the context of a significant lack of administrative and legislative capacity, with inspiration from foreign healthcare legislation.[24] Recalling the making of the plans for the new insurance system, one of the participants at the Ministry of Health said:

> While there was a huge enthusiasm about the reform, nobody knew how specific mechanisms would work in practice….Even the health insurance system—we did not really know how to put it in law—so we asked the

[23] Interview No. 10.
[24] Interview No. 10.

mother of one of our colleagues who spoke German to translate some parts of the German insurance law and then we integrated that in the reform plan.[25]

Previous strict adherence to the socialist health policy paradigm meant the policymakers had no experience with forms of healthcare system organisation other than those within a state-dominated, centralised, and bureaucratic system. Therefore, when the communist regime collapsed, even though there was general agreement on the deficiencies of the socialist system, 'there was no widespread understanding of what exactly the market-oriented health reform would entail'.[26]

Despite the unfavourable policy legacy, the Ministerial team under Pithart's government prepared a set of bills defining the functioning of the new insurance system: Bill on General Health Insurance, Bill on the General Health Insurance Fund, and Bill on Departmental, Professional, Corporate and other Health Insurance Funds. The first bill introduced a compulsory health insurance based on payroll contributions set at 13.5 per cent of workers' wages, 4.5 per cent of which would be paid by the employee and 9 per cent by the employer. The government would pay contributions for workers' dependents and the unemployed, whilst the self-employed would be obliged to pay the entire premium, calculated as 13.5 per cent of 35 per cent of their income before taxation. This bill also specified fee-for-service based on a points system as the main reimbursement method for services delivered in both primary and secondary care.

The second bill established the General Health Insurance Fund (GHIF), and the third called for the establishment of additional health insurance funds (HIFs). According to the third bill, any population group of 50,000 could set up its own insurance fund. Each of these funds would be required to cover services from the government's package of defined health benefits and pay for them using the fee-for-service scheme, as this was defined in additional legislation.[27] The bill introduced a competitive element in the system allowing HIFs to offer benefits in addition to the basic benefit package. The main idea was that competition between the HIFs and the GHIF would concentrate not only on the quality of services offered but also on the provision of additional benefits to clients. Competition was additionally fostered by the provision that the HIFs could derive savings

[25] Interview No. 10.
[26] Interview No. 9.
[27] Decree 467/1992.

by negotiating lower prices within the fee-for-service scheme with physicians and hospitals. As a final incentive for competition, an HIF's clients would be able to change to another HIF, if they wished, every six months (Scheffler 1999). Once up for parliamentary discussion, the three bills passed easily in Parliament, given the government's strong majority.[28]

Regulation of Competition

As mentioned earlier in the chapter, the June 1992 elections were crucial for the crystallisation of some of the country's key political forces and marked the formation of party divisions on the traditional left-right axis (Mansfeldová 2013: 222). One of the main fractions of the Civic Forum, the ODS, was the most successful competitor in the electoral run, winning almost 30 per cent of the votes. The 1992 elections also saw the parliamentary debut of the ČSSD, as it passed the electoral threshold and gained 16 seats. The government was formed by the ODS in coalition with four other parties: KDS, ODA, and a coalition of KDU and ČSL. The coalition government held 105 out of 200 seats in Parliament and was led by Klaus as Prime Minister. Despite this slim majority, the coalition survived the full term, facing down the transitional turmoil and, as it will be shown, dramatically failed health reform.

The Klaus government had to tackle some major political issues, including the dissolution of the federal state and the large-scale restructuring of the Czech economy. Yet, implementation of the health insurance system became one of the government's major headaches. Soon after the above bills were passed, 27 HIFs emerged in the insurance market, taking over a significant share of clients from the GHIF (Vepřek et al. 2002; Bryndová et al. 2019). The competition between the GHIF and the HIFs developed quickly, and the new insurance system was plunged into a serious crisis. The main issue was the problem of spiralling costs. The open-ended fee-for-service reimbursement scheme based on a point system motivated healthcare providers to overproduce services, thus stimulating supply-induced demand, which, in turn, drained resources from the insurance funds.

[28] *Zákon o všeobecném zdravotním pojištění*, Law No. 550/1991; *Zákon o Všeobecné zdravotní pojišťovně*, Law No. 551/1991; *Zákon o resortních, oborových, podnikových a dalších zdravotních pojišťovnách*, Law No. 280/1992.

Another cause of the failure of the insurance system was open competition. The tendency of HIFs to create special insurance packages attractive to young and healthy citizens generated market failures in the form of adverse selection and cream skimming, leaving the GHIF with a small number of insured individuals and a disproportionate share of the elderly with more complex healthcare needs (Bryndová et al. 2019).[29] As later analysis revealed, under the fee-for-service scheme, it was common for physicians to bill for more than 100 hours per week. Meanwhile, private surgeons billed for over 25 per cent more points than those in the public hospitals. The annual budget of the GHIF was nearly depleted in the first six months of the fiscal year. Many of the private funds had even more severe financial problems, as they fell into insolvency and were declared bankrupt, so that their clients had to be taken over by the GHIF. The cumulative debt of the GHIF increased, reaching roughly 10 million Czech crowns (Scheffler 1999).

With the crisis of the healthcare sector looming large, Minister of Health Luděk Rubáš admitted it was a mistake to introduce open competition in the health insurance market without a properly functioning insurance system in place (ČTK 1995a). To tackle the crisis, the Ministry amended the 1991 Law on General Health Insurance Fund and introduced controls for the fee-for-service scheme. The Ministry of Finance, in consultation with the Ministry of Health, would set the maximum price of the points based on the proposal of the insurance fund.[30] A second amendment introduced regulations of the insurance market that involved, among others, supervision and regular audits of the HIFs and not allowing HIFs to offer additional insurance benefits.[31] Interestingly, even though Parliament accepted these measures, with the strong support of the Ministry of Finance, the ČSSD opposed them, arguing the regulation of competition would lead to a monopoly in the hands of the public GHIF (ČTK 1995b). Whilst this could be understood as an opposition party's way to point to the failures of the government's reforms, it also suggested the ČSSD was working on solidifying its social-democratic identity to clearly distinguish itself from the old communists.

[29] The extra benefits of their insurance package included free travel insurance or subsidies for wellness activities (Bryndová et al. 2019), thus revealing the intentions of the funds to attract younger and healthier clients.

[30] Amendment to the Law on General Health Insurance, Law No. 59/1995.

[31] Amendment to the Law on General Health Insurance, Law No. 60/1995.

Not surprisingly, Czech doctors did not like the limits imposed on fees-for-service. Their dissatisfaction built on a more general hostility to the Ministry of Health; they repeatedly accused Minister Rubáš of trying to reduce professional power through changes in medical licensing and the abolition of obligatory membership in the Medical Chamber. The disagreement grew as doctors opposed more specific measures proposed by the Minister to contain costs. For example, Rubáš wanted to introduce a referral system that would assign an important role to general practitioners (GPs), and he proposed a small user fee for specialist visits without a GP referral. However, this idea went against the interests of the specialists who preferred to maximise the fee-for-service scheme and thus refused to support anything contrary to it (ČTK 1995c).

Hoping to smooth things over, Minister Rubáš initiated a dialogue between healthcare professionals, unions, and health insurance funds and established a tripartite body called 'Consultation Committee for Health Policy'. However, the working of this Committee was obstructed by a deepening difference of opinion between the Ministry and the doctors. At the same time, the government tried to profit from the split among professionals, as evidenced in the emergence of new professional group, Doctor's Trade Union Club (*Lékařský Odborový Klub—Svaz Českýh Lékařů—LOK—SČL*) in March 1995. Rubáš started negotiating with LOK and ignored the other two professional organisations—the Medical Chamber and the Health and Social Care Trade Union. The latter two joined the opposition's calls for Rubáš' resignation, and the LOK followed them. Seeing no progress in the dialogue, the Ministry decided to suspend the Committee's meetings. Things went from bad to worse, as this resulted in a series of medical strikes (Potůček 1999: 92).

The regulations introduced by the 1995 amendments were only partly helpful in solving the problems of the insurance sector, as the sector continued to generate financial deficits. The ineffective reaction of the government, according to one expert, could be traced to the Ministry's refusal to recognise the causes of particular failures within the system (see also Háva and Kružík 1995).[32] Rubáš's conflicts with doctors and his inability to end the crisis generated calls for his resignation, and Prime Minister Klaus replaced him with Jan Stráský.

In his reform plan submitted to Parliament, Stráský took advantage of proposals prepared during Rubáš's term, the Short-Term and the

[32] Interview No. 11.

Long-Term Programme (Ministry of Health 1995a, b). The Short-Term Programme proposed cost-saving measures, including the introduction of selective contracting, changes in reimbursement methods, gatekeeping, and co-payments. The Long-Term Programme was more radical, as it proposed dividing the healthcare system into two tiers: one would be public, solidarity-based health insurance, and the other would be an individual medical savings account.

The Long-Term Programme was shelved immediately, as it was rejected by the coalition of Christian democrats (KDU-ČSL), which represented the second largest party in the government coalition. The discussion of the measures proposed in the Short-Term Program was also stalled, as it encountered opposition from doctors, despite renewed attempts to reach agreement through social dialogue. In fact, this was doomed to fail—the government saw dialogue as unnecessary claiming healthcare was its responsibility (ČTK 1996).

Turning to a more urgent issue, the continuously growing deficit in the insurance sector, Stráský's Ministry introduced further amendments to the Law on General Health Insurance to better regulate the insurance sector. These measures included the definition of procedures for liquidation, mergers of health insurance funds, and a provision whereby the remaining HIFs would be supervised by the Ministry of Health and Finance and obliged to provide regular financial reports. Other important measures were the introduction of a risk-adjustment scheme which would redistribute revenues of the insurance funds according to the age structure of their clients[33] and the establishment of a Reserve Fund to settle outstanding payables in the case of fund bankruptcies. To regulate competition, under the new measures, the HIFs could be changed every 12 months.[34] The overall effect of the regulation measures was quickly visible, as the number of insurance funds began to decrease through liquidation or mergers of smaller and less efficient funds (Vepřek et al. 2002).

Whilst a combination of regulation and a lack of incentives for competition stabilised the insurance sector, the overproduction of health services stimulated by the fee-for-service scheme was still posing risks for the financial solvency of the healthcare sector. Final efforts to regulate the Czech

[33] Initially, only 60 per cent of the revenues were redistributed. This mechanism was refined in 2005, introducing the redistribution of all health insurance system revenues based on age and gender (Bryndová et al. 2019).

[34] Amendment to the Law on General Health Insurance, Law No. 149/1996.

healthcare market occurred with the change in the political constellation after the 1996 elections. The highlight of these elections, the first held after the breakup of the federal state, was the emergence of the ČSSD as a serious rival to the previously dominant ODS (Mansfeldová 2013: 225). In a major improvement from the 1992 elections, the ČSSD quadrupled its electoral support and received more than a quarter of all votes. Yet, as the ČSSD was unwilling to align with the communists and unable to find another suitable coalition partner, the ODS again formed a government with three of its previous allies (the ODA and the KDU-ČSL coalition). However, as the combined strength of the parties of the ODS coalition amounted to only 99 out of 200 seats, government formation depended on the approval of the opposition parties, particularly the ČSSD. The ČSSD informally agreed to support the government in exchange for important leadership positions on parliamentary committees and the appointment of the party head Miloš Zeman as Chairman of the Chamber of Deputies (Bugajski 2002: 38).

One of the leadership positions given to the ČSSD was the role of the head of the parliamentary Committee for Social Policy and Health. This was given to Vladimír Špidla. With a party member in this position, the ČSSD could shape the healthcare legislation of the new government. Moreover, whilst the ODS kept Stráský as the head of the Ministry of Health, the new government, again led by Klaus, passed a substantive change that ended the competition in healthcare provision. The 1997 Law on Public Health Insurance[35] replaced the 1991 Law on General Health Insurance. It integrated elements of the previous legislation that aimed at regulating the insurance sector, but the most important addition was the replacement of the competitive fee-for-service scheme with a mix of fee-for-service and capitation in primary care and budget-based payment in hospital care.[36] The law also introduced selective contracting between healthcare providers and insurance funds and defined the volume limits in contracts, thus more strictly controlling the relationship between funds and healthcare providers.

The parliamentary debate on the law demonstrated the ČSSD party's focus on the regulation of the health sector and its political influence during the preparation of the reform. This was evident in Špidla's role as

[35] *Zákon o verejném zdravotním pojistení*, Law No. 48/1997.

[36] The law kept fee-for-service for ambulatory specialists, but set a uniform point value negotiated between insurance funds and providers and approved by the Ministry of Finance.

rapporteur for the 1997 law. Moreover, during the final parliamentary discussion, all ČSSD MPs voted for it (Chamber of Deputies of the Czech Republic 1997).[37]

However, the party took a softer stance on the government's market-oriented approach; it made concessions to some liberal elements in the law, such as the distinction between the 'standard' and 'non-standard' care, with a stipulation that only the former would be covered by public health insurance, and also to the increase in co-payments for health services defined as 'non-essential' (Bryndová et al. 2019: 38; Jaroš and Kalina 1998).

Despite the ČSSD's concessions, the main aim of regulating the healthcare market was achieved. The measures introduced in the 1997 law quickly produced tangible results, most visible in the dramatic reduction in the number of health insurance funds (down to nine) and the relative stabilisation of the insurance sector. Yet, the GHIF continued to grow its deficit, mainly because in contrast to the other funds, it was obliged to cover the unemployed, whose insurance contributions were funded by the state (Vepřek et al. 2002). In the future, this led to a series of measures to reduce the deficit, including the clearing of GHIF debts through the Czech Consolidation Agency in 2002 and, in the context of the global financial crisis, the 2013 emergency measures granting the GHIF a government loan worth 1.7 billion Czech crowns (Alexa et al. 2015: 46).

Privatisation of Primary Care

Another key episode of market reform in the first post-communist decade involved privatisation of primary care. The law introducing privatisation was passed under the Pithart government and, like the insurance legislation, was based on the proposal prepared by Health Minister's Bojar reform team led by Kamil Kalina. Passed as the 1992 Law on Healthcare in Non-State Healthcare Facilities, this law allowed private forms of healthcare delivery in both outpatient and inpatient care, specifying conditions of operation for non-state, that is, private healthcare facilities.[38] The passing of this law took place in the political context still marked by the conflict between communists and non-communists; it easily passed in Parliament given the majority of the non-communist Civic Forum.

[37] Only the MPs belonging to the communist successor party (KSČM) opposed the law.

[38] *Zákon o zdravotní péči v nestátních zdravotnických zařízeních*, Law No. 160/1992.

While the 1992 law explicitly opened the door for privatisation of primary care, once again, there were some implementation hiccups. The privatisation process was delegated to the Ministry of Privatisation, especially established for this purpose, and to the National Property Fund; thus, the Ministry of Health was excluded from a process that involved making decisions on which specific healthcare facilities would be available for privatisation. This led to a conflict between the two Ministries, as they disagreed over the scope of privatisation. The Ministry of Health objected to the privatisation list of the Ministry of Privatisation, arguing it contained serious mistakes; some healthcare facilities were unaccounted for and others were erroneously earmarked for privatisation. This generated a delay in approval of the list of healthcare facilities for privatisation and more generally resulted in confusion. Three months after the passage of the 1992 law, the government approved a list of facilities for privatisation and extended the deadline for submission of privatisation projects by another three months (Háva and Kružík 1995).

In practice, implementation of healthcare delivery privatisation took two main forms. One included transfer of former polyclinics to communities or towns and their subsequent division into single practices, which then became available for rent by private physicians. Another form was used mainly for privatisation of ambulatory care and involved direct privatisation of the buildings of the polyclinics, which then became available for rent by a group of physicians or another party. Despite the decision-making hiccups, the privatisation model using these two methods was quite successful. It resulted in the quick and almost complete privatisation of outpatient care—95 per cent of Czech primary care physicians provided their services privately by the mid-1990s (Scheffler 1999).

Introduction of User Fees

At the beginning of the second post-socialist decade, Czech healthcare policy was marked with absence of major reforms. The 1998 elections witnessed the first post-communist victory of the social democratic ČSSD party. After weeks of negotiations with potential coalition partners, the ČSSD decided to form a one-party minority government with the formal support of the ODS through an 'opposition agreement' (Kopecký 2007; Mansfeldová 2013).[39] The cooperation between the two parties was not a new thing; it had started in 1996 when the ČSSD agreed to informally support the minority government led by the ODS. The ODS's decision to do the same in 1998 could thus be interpreted as a return of political favours (see Bugajski 2002), but this time, the cooperation was formalised, suggesting their ideological differences were more moderate than it might seem. The period of the ČSSD minority government was indeed marked by mass public protests criticising the parties' cooperation and pointing to the 'collusion of ODS and ČSSD', suggesting a lack of clear political alternatives (Dvořáková 2003; see also Kopecký 2007).

The moderation of differences between the ODS and the ČSSD was further confirmed by the government formation after the 2002 elections. Winning the elections but again falling short of the number of seats needed for a parliamentary majority, the ČSSD decided to form a government with the ODS's previous coalition partner, the pro-social but also pro-market Christian democratic coalition, the KDU-ČSL, and with the small liberal party, Freedom Union (US-DEU). The ČSSD's decision to enter a coalition with these two instead of the old communists (KSČM), although the latter union would ensure a comfortable majority in Parliament, suggested its clear preference for positioning itself closer to the political centre. Whilst this alliance seemed to bring the ČSSD closer to the ODS, however, the ODS-ČSSD ideological differences in health policy became evident during the next major episode of healthcare reform, this one involving user fees.

During the 2006 election campaign, the ODS presented a new plan for the reform of the health system. This plan was prepared by a group of experts gathered around an organisation called Forum for Czech Health Reform (*Fórum pro reformu českého zdravotnictví*), and published as 'Healthcare Reform in the Czech Republic in 21st Century Europe' (Hroboň et al. 2005). This 100-page document proposed large-scale reform involving three major measures: hospital privatisation, re-establishment of managed competition in the insurance sector, and introduction of user fees. After the ODS won the elections and formed a government in summer 2006, it used this document as the basis for the

[39] The official title was: 'Agreement on Creating a Stable Political Environment in the Czech Republic concluded between the Czech Social Democratic Party (ČSSD) and the Civic Democratic Party (ODS)' (Mansfeldová 2013: 238).

government's official plan for health reform. However, the government's zeal for large-scale reform was not matched by its strength—the ODS formed a government alone in a minority configuration led by Mirek Topolánek. The government was reshuffled in January 2007, in an attempt to strengthen it by adding the ODS's old political ally, the KDU-ČSL and the Green Party (SZ). This was not entirely successful, however, as the three parties together held exactly half of the parliamentary seats, casting doubt on the possibility of major reform.

Topolánek signalled his determination to push for large-scale health reform by appointing Tomáš Julínek as Minister of Health. Julínek was an ODS member and a former senator, but more importantly, he was one of the authors of the ODS reform proposal published during the election campaign.[40] Shortly after entering office, Julínek used this document to prepare an official government proposal for reform. After the government entered a coalition with the KDU-ČSL and SZ, it became clear that the major coalition partner (KDU-ČSL) was not in favour of it, so Julínek decided to scale down his Ministry's reform ambition by concentrating on user fees as the reform's main aspect. Apart from being political, the decision to abandon the large-scale plan and focus on user fees was also strategic, as Julínek and his team thought it would be easier to build consensus around a relatively simple reform that did not require major legislative changes—just a few additional paragraphs in the existing law.[41]

Yet, the decision proved risky, as user fees became a hotly debated issue. This debate over the introduction of the fees as one form of patient payment for healthcare services echoed the political dispute in the mid-1990s when patient payments for healthcare services were publicly controversial. In 1995, the Klaus government proposed changes in patient payments in an attempt to save the healthcare system from plunging further into the crisis caused by the failures of the managed competition reform. The plan was to contain costs by increasing the co-payments and introducing user fees. This triggered a prolonged parliamentary debate between the ODS and the ČSSD. The dispute even led to the Constitutional Court whose ruling determined the introduction of patient co-payments for basic healthcare services violated the constitutional right to healthcare (Czech Constitutional Court 1995).

[40] Interview No. 16.
[41] Interview No. 12.

This renewed attempt to private healthcare costs through user fees did not start off well, as the government discovered it lacked support even within its own ranks. As mentioned above, the second Topolánek government was formed by the ODS in a coalition with the KDU–ČSL and the Greens. Almost immediately, the KDU–ČSL started to criticise the Ministry's proposal, and the Greens, as the third coalition partner, followed suit. This significantly weakened the chances that the proposal would get parliamentary support, as the ODS needed its partners' votes. Aware that the introduction of the fees could be a tough nut to crack, Julínek's Ministry organised a series of meetings with representatives of all parliamentary parties and a group of healthcare experts. The main aim of these meetings, called 'Round Tables on Healthcare Reform', was to try to build consensus around the Ministry's reform plan. However, there was never any real debate on the reform, as Julínek kept a hard stance, at one point even entering into a heated discussion with the ČSSD representatives, prompting the latter to leave the negotiations.[42]

The ODS was left alone, so it sought support from healthcare professionals, only to hit another wall. Interestingly, Czech doctors opposed the introduction of user fees, even though these direct payments would lead to an immediate increase in their income. The doctors felt receiving direct payments from patients would be reminiscent of the corruption during communism, thus interfering with their relationships with their patients. Instead of user fees, they preferred increasing their pay by making changes in the existing reimbursement schemes.[43]

Facing strong opposition, the ODS realised its policy proposal, even if it passed, would be most likely dismissed by the Constitutional Court given the Court's clear stance on the unconstitutionality of user fees expressed in its 1995 ruling. Surprisingly, however, the party reached its policy aims. Its eventual success drew on an exceptional strategy that allowed the party to circumvent the potential vetoes. Acknowledging that seeking further compromises with either KDU-ČSL or ČSSD would probably be futile, the ODS made a strategic move—it integrated user fees into a proposal for a Law on Public Budget Stabilisation.[44] This law presented user fees not as major change to the existing model of healthcare provision but as a necessary fiscal measure to stabilise the state budget.

[42] Interview No. 12.
[43] Interview No. 13.
[44] *Zákon o stabilizaci veřejných rozpočtů*, Law No. 261/2007.

Specifically, the need to stabilise the public budget was justified by claim that the country had to adopt fiscal policies that would align its macroeconomic conditions with the rest of the European Union, to which it now belonged.

Interestingly, in the text of the law, user fees for medical services were termed 'regulatory fees' (*regulační poplatky*), and their main aim was interpreted as a measure to avoid the abuse of services that would also help regulate healthcare spending. During the parliamentary discussion, this wording was vehemently criticised by the ČSSD (Rath 2006). The reframing of the reform in terms of fiscal concerns and regulative measures convinced the KDU-ČSL, however; the party put fiscal concerns first and voted in support of the law. It was passed with a slim majority, including the votes of the government MPs and additional votes from the independents (Chamber of Deputies of the Czech Republic 2007).

The introduced fees amounted to 30 crowns (equivalent to €1.20) for a doctor's visit and for every item on a drug prescription, 60 crowns (€2.40) for a day in hospital, 90 crowns (€3.60) for a visit by ambulatory services outside office hours and for an emergency treatment (van Ginneken et al. 2010). The law also granted exemptions from fees for specific population groups, such as those living below the poverty line, children, pregnant women, and patients with infectious diseases. In addition, it introduced an annual ceiling of 5000 crowns (€200) per insured individual, which excluded fees for hospital stays and fees for the use of ambulatory services outside office hours. Above this limit, further user fees would be reimbursed by the insurance funds (Bryndová et al. 2019).

As expected, the ČSSD immediately brought the newly instituted fees to the Constitutional Court, arguing they went against the constitutional provision of free healthcare provision and posed a major threat to patients' access to health services. Yet, the Court seemed to buy into the ODS's justification logic, ruling the fees should be retained as they represented an integral component of the government's plan to balance the state budget. The Court also determined they did not constitute a real threat to healthcare access (Czech Constitutional Court 2008).

Encouraged by the success of his policy manoeuvring, Minister Julínek tried to resuscitate his original plan for large-scale reform, but this attempt was quickly obstructed by the strong opposition of the ODS's coalition partners, the KDU-ČSL and the Greens. In the meantime, the user fees became increasingly unpopular among the public. Czechs were not really bothered by the relatively small amount of the fees, but they understandably did not like paying for what used to be free healthcare delivery (Antonova et al. 2010). The fees became a heated issue in the upcoming regional and Senate elections, with the ČSSD pledging to abolish fees in regional hospitals and pharmacies if the party won (van Ginneken et al. 2010). As the ČSSD won both elections, the fees became even more controversial, motivating Topolanek to replace Julínek with Daniela Filipiová.

Partial Withdrawal of User Fees

As it had gained power in all regions in the elections, the ČSSD started to fight against the fees on a local level. In February 2009, the regional governments decided the fees for medical services would be paid from the regional budgets. This new measure encountered various difficulties in implementation, however. In some regions, patients were automatically reimbursed, whilst in others, they had to fill in a written request, causing administrative problems (van Ginneken et al. 2010). Public pharmacies but not private ones were able to use regional budgets to reimburse patients. Private pharmacies lost customers and appealed to the High Court. They won their case: the Court prohibited the reimbursements on the grounds of unfair competition (IDNES 2009). As a countermeasure, the ČSSD responded by threatening to appeal to the Constitutional Court (IDNES 2010a).

The issue of user fees even gained the attention of the European Union, with the European Commission arguing the regional authorities' reimbursements were discriminatory. The Commission also said that if the reimbursement of fees were formally investigated, this policy risked being found at odds with the EU's state-aid rules (ČTK 2010). Another problem was that the reimbursements placed a great burden on regional budgets; after only one year of implementation the cost equalled 478 million Czech crowns, about 19 million euros (van Ginneken et al. 2010).

Topolanek's government fell in spring 2009, torn by internal frictions and adversely affected by the controversy swirling around the user fees. It was replaced by a caretaker government led by Jan Fischer. Facing difficulties in its fight against the user fees at the regional level, the ČSSD continued its struggle in Parliament, obtaining a small victory by eliminating the fee for a doctor's visit for children below 18 years of age and lowering the cap on the annual ceiling for both children and the elderly (those over

65 years of age) from 5000 to 2500 crowns.[45] However, as it still lacked the votes it needed to completely abolish the fees, the party admitted it had lost the fight and would try again after the next elections (IDNES 2010b).

Yet, even though the ČSSD was the frontrunner in the 2010 elections, the ODS formed a strong majority government in a coalition with two political newcomers, the conservative Tradition, Responsibility, Prosperity (*Tradice Odpovědnost Prosperita*—TOP09) and the liberal Public Affairs (*Věci veřejné*—VV) under Petr Nečas. The results of the 2010 elections, dominated by the global financial crisis, were generally seen a surprise, as both ODS and ČSSD lost substantial support (Hanley 2012). The relative strength of the new political forces in the Nečas government was indicated by the appointment of Leoš Heger from TOP09 as the Minister of Health.

Justifying the move as an attempt to offset the effects of the global financial crisis,[46] in 2011, the Nečas government increased the fee for a day in hospital from 60 to 100 crowns (€2.20).[47] At the same time, the Ministry of Health created a list of items belonging to 'above-standard' care.[48] This list was relatively short and included some types of vaccinations, plasters, and artificial eye lenses. It was meant to enable patients to choose between standard and above-standard treatment; to get better artificial eye lenses, for example, a patient would pay the difference between the superior and the standard treatment. The Ministry pointed out that in the existing system, patients had to pay the full cost of the more expensive treatment, unless it was prescribed for a specific medical reason, in which case it was covered by the insurance system. According to Minister Heger, this practice nurtured informal patient payments to doctors, and the aim of the 'above-standard' list was to eliminate these (Alexa et al. 2015: 124).

The ČSSD attacked these two measures, appealing to the Constitutional Court on the grounds that the increase in hospital fees threatened access to healthcare for vulnerable groups. It also contested the division between standard and above-standard care. In July 2013, the Court ruled this increase was unfair to vulnerable groups, and the hospital fee must be

[45] Amendment to the Law on Public Health Insurance, Law No. 59/2009. Through another amendment to the 1997 laws, in 2017, the amount of 2500 crowns was further reduced to 1000 crowns (Law No. 290/2017).

[46] Interview No. 19.

[47] Amendments to the Law on Public Health Insurance, Law No. 298/2011 and Law No. 369/2011.

[48] Decree No. 411/2011.

abolished from 1 January 2014. Interestingly, in its 2008 ruling, the Court had supported the introduction of fees, but it now argued that the fee for a hospital visit was basically a 'payment for hotel services'. The Court also ruled against the division between standard and above-standard care based on the difficulties involved in interpreting the actual difference between the two types of care (Czech Constitutional Court 2013).

The remaining user fees stayed in place until 2014. The ČSSD won the 2013 elections and thus ended the eight-year rule of the ODS. It formed a government with the KDU-ČSL and a new political force, the liberal ANO under Bohuslav Sobotka. Interestingly, however, the healthcare law introduced under this ČSSD government did not abolish the fees altogether, but reduced them to 30 crowns and retained the 90-crown fee for emergency services.[49]

The ČSSD's reluctance to fully reverse the user fee reform could be attributed to its coalition with the liberal ANO, but also to the fact that fiscal concerns started to play a more important role in the government's policymaking in the aftermath of the global financial crisis, something demonstrated by the appointment of ANO's leader Andrej Babiš as the Minister of Finance in Sobotka's government (Hanley and Vachudova 2018).[50] Whilst the decision to keep the fees within the legislative framework could be seen as a combination of political and fiscal factors, it also suggested the ČSSD's position on healthcare reforms was significantly shaped by the political dynamics and thus open for compromise.

Hospital Privatisation

The last major episode of market-oriented healthcare reforms in the Czech Republic revolved around a long-disputed issue of hospital transformation. The question of change in hospital ownership emerged in the early 1990s, when the 1992 Law on Healthcare in Non-State Healthcare Facilities allowed the privatisation of healthcare delivery. Although the privatisation of primary care during this period went relatively smoothly, hospital privatisation became a hot issue. The 1992 law allowed the privatisation of both outpatient and inpatient care, which implied hospitals could be privatised, but the law did not specify the exact form of

[49] Amendments to the Law on Public Health Insurance, Law No. 256/2014.

[50] During its electoral campaign, ANO promised Babiš would run the state 'efficiently' like a business (Havlík 2015).

privatisation. As the government's implementation process lacked clearly established guidelines, various models of hospital privatisation became extensively debated (Háva and Kružík 1995).

One of the major issues was the lack of a legal form of ownership that would be suitable for hospitals in contrast to, for example, former state-owned industrial enterprises that could easily be privatised under the existing legal framework. Another issue was which hospitals should be privatised. Some were teaching hospitals that trained physicians and other health professionals, and many were involved in clinical and biomedical research. Given their important public functions, trade unions and health-care professionals argued they should not be up for privatisation, so these hospitals were taken off the privatisation list.[51] Another more practical issue was that the majority of public hospitals were in dire financial straits and thus offered no incentives to private investors.[52] As a result, hospital privatisation was stalled, and only about 10 small private hospitals with fewer than 2000 beds, or three per cent of total hospital capacity, were privatised by the end of the 1990s (Jaroš et al. 2005: 223).

The new phase of hospital reform was preceded by the large-scale reform of public administration introduced in 1997 by the Constitutional Law on the Establishment of Higher Territorial Self-Governing Units.[53] This law, passed under the ODS government, decentralised the existing public administration structure by dividing the country into 14 regions and transferred the ownership of approximately half of the Czech hospitals to the newly formed regions. After the transfer, faced with chronic deficits in some of the hospitals, the regions decided to change their legal form, transforming them from organisations subordinate to the regional authorities to joint-stock companies. This implied they would operate according to laws on private ownership and would thus be able to make a profit, even though regions or lower administrative units, such as districts or municipalities, would be their major shareholders. This change was important: whilst hospitals would initially remain publicly owned, in the future they could, as commercial companies, be sold to private investors (Mihalco 2007).

By 2000, hospital transformation was underway, but the government, now led by the ČSSD, attempted to use its parliamentary powers to block

[51] Interview No. 8.
[52] Interview No. 14.
[53] *Ústavní zákon o vytvoření vyšších územních samosprávných celků*, Law. No. 347/1997.

it. In the policy debate, the old communists (KSČM) sided with the ČSSD arguing against the transformation. In 2005, the ČSSD government, with support from the KSČM, tried to prevent the change in hospital ownership by amending the Law on the Protection of Public Health[54] to prohibit territorial self-governing units from converting medical facilities into commercial companies. These amendments were vetoed by the Senate and the President (ČTK 2005). This was expected, as the ODS and KDU-ČSL held a majority in the Upper House, and the President was ODS leader Václav Klaus. The Presidential veto was overturned in Parliament, and the law was passed again, with the support of the KSČM (Chamber of Deputies of the Czech Republic 2005).

The ČSSD's efforts to prevent hospital transformation culminated in 2006, with the passing of the Law on Public Non-Profit Healthcare Facilities.[55] This law aimed to prevent hospitals from becoming joint-stock companies by stipulating that 140 district hospitals would be transformed into non-profit hospitals and put under the direct supervision of the Ministry of Health. During the parliamentary debate, the ODS criticised the law arguing it represented significant interference in property rights and the performance of the self-governing function of the regions. Above all, it did not contribute to the solution of the problems of the healthcare sector (Langer 2002). The ČSSD's Minister of Health David Rath remained firm, arguing that shifting hospitals' status to non-profit was necessary to prevent them from becoming regular money-making businesses and then privatised (Rath 2006). Ultimately, Parliament passed the law with the backing of the ČSSD and the KSČM (Chamber of Deputies of the Czech Republic 2006a).

Both the Senate and the President again returned the law to Parliament. Klaus' veto, was clearly supportive of his party's stance on the issue, but the veto was overridden, as the ČSSD and the KSČM again voted for it (Chamber of Deputies of the Czech Republic 2006b). The ODS was not willing to give up, however, and it appealed to the Constitutional Court arguing the law was unconstitutional because it violated the ownership rights of lower administrative units and introduced unequal conditions for different health providers. The Court determined that some of the law's provisions were indeed unconstitutional as they interfered with

[54] Amendments to the Law on the Protection of Public Health (Law No. 258/2000), Law No. 392/2005.

[55] *Zákon o veřejných neziskových ústavních zdravotnických zařízeních*, Law No. 245/2006.

constitutional property rights and rights of self-government. The Court's ruling more specifically stated that the law constituted a fundamental incursion into the healthcare competence of the territorial units as it forced these units to change the legal form of healthcare facilities and subordinated them to the Ministry of Health. The Court concluded that the hospitals should be left to decide on their own whether they wanted to convert to a non-profit status (Constitutional Court 2006).

The ČSSD's efforts to block hospital transformation were reversed in 2011, when the ODS-led majority government repealed the 2006 law and nullified the 2005 amendments.[56] The regions were given free range to transform hospitals into joint stock companies and sell their shares to private investors. As a result, by 2018, 98 Czech hospitals were registered as private, compared to 158 registered as public (OECD 2020). These hospitals remain under public ownership, since regional authorities are majority shareholders, but act under private law.

Conclusion

This chapter has provided an empirical account of health reforms in post-communist Czech Republic. This country established a system of social health insurance in which private health insurance plays a marginal role, but primary and, increasingly, hospital care are delivered privately. The analysis suggested this public–private mix was the result of rather bumpy policy path characterised by significant *instability* and hence markedly different from Slovenia's and Poland's policy trajectories of *survival* and *reversal*, respectively, of market reforms. The chapter accounted for the origins of the Czech post-communist health reforms by querying the health policy under socialism. It showed how the emergence of market ideas combined with a lack of actual experience with policies other than those based on the centralised Soviet healthcare model inspired radical reform choices in post-communism that led to textbook examples of market failure. The subsequent policy developments were shaped by the country's unique political and institutional arrangements, including moderate party divisions, marked by both conflicts and pragmatic compromises, and judicial vetoes. The result was a trial and error process of policy learning, wherein market policies were tested in repeated and strategic reform attempts, with varying success.

[56] Law No. 466/2011.

References

Alexa, Jan, Lukáš Rečka, Jana Votápková, Ewout van Ginneken, Anne Spranger, and Friedrich Wittenbecher. 2015. Czech Republic: Health system review. WHO Regional Office for Europe, European Observatory on Healthcare Systems and Policies.

Antonova, Petra, Daniel Jacobs, Martin Bojar, Rudolf Rudolf Černý, Katerina Ciharová, Melissa A. Frick, Bara Fintel, Jack DeHovitz, and Charles L. Bennett. 2010. Czech health two decades on from the Velvet Revolution. *Lancet* 375 (9710): 179–181.

Bryndová, Lucie, Kateřina Pavloková, Tomáš Roubal, Martina Rokosová, and Matthew Gaskins. 2019. Czech Republic: Health system review. WHO Regional Office for Europe, European Observatory on Healthcare Systems and Policies.

Bugajski, Janusz. 2002. *Political parties of Eastern Europe: A guide to politics in the post-communist era*. Armonk, NY and London: Sharpe.

Cabada, Ladislav. 2010. Traditional, third way or a different path? The Czech Social Democrat Party in 2010. *Politics in Central Europe* 6 (1): 83–89.

Calda, Miloš. 1996. The Roundtable Talks in Czechoslovakia. In *The Roundtable Talks and the breakdown of communism*, ed. Jon Elster, 135–177. Chicago: University of Chicago Press.

Casal Bértoa, Fernando. 2011. Sources of party system institutionalization in new democracies: Lessons from East Central Europe. EUI SPS Working Paper 2011/01, Cadmus, EUI Research Repository. http://hdl.handle.net/1814/15804.

———. 2014. Party systems and cleavage structures revisited: A sociological explanation of party system institutionalization in East Central Europe. *Party Politics* 20 (1): 16–36.

Chamber of Deputies of the Czech Republic. 1997. Voting for the Law on Public Health Insurance (Law No. 48/1997). https://www.psp.cz/sqw/hlasy.sqw?G=8497. Accessed 20 March 2022.

———. 2005. Voting for the Amendments to the Law on the Protection of Public Health (Law No. 258/2000), Law No. 392/2005. https://psp.cz/sqw/hlasy.sqw?G=39878. Accessed 25 March 2022.

———. 2006a. First voting on the Law on Public Non-Profit Healthcare Facilities (Law No. 245/2006). https://www.psp.cz/sqw/hlasy.sqw?G=42728. Accessed 25 March 2022.

———. 2006b. Second voting on the Law on Public Non-Profit Healthcare Facilities (Law No. 245/2006). https://www.psp.cz/sqw/hlasy.sqw?G=43549. Accessed 25 March 2022.

———. 2007. Voting on the Law on Public Budget Stabilization (Law No. 261/2007). https://www.psp.cz/sqw/hlasy.sqw?G=45638. Accessed 25 March 2022.

Charter 77. 1984. *Zdraví je součastí práva na život.* Praha, Charta 77, dok. č.14/84 z 15. srpna 1984. Listy, Časopis československé socialistické opozice, Příloha k č. 6, 1984. http://scriptum.cz/soubory//scriptum/listy rim/listy_1984_6_priloha_zm_ocr.pdf. Accessed 10 March 2022.

Constitution of the Czech Republic. 1993. https://www.psp.cz/en/docs/laws/1993/1.html. Accessed 5 March 2022.

Czech Constitutional Court. 1995. PI.ÚS 35/95. http://kraken.slv.cz/Pl.US35/95. Accessed 17 March 2022.

———. 2006. Pl ÚS 51/06. https://www.usoud.cz/en/decisions/20060927-pl-us-5106-non-profit-hospitals1/?mediaid=1568737&title=episod-5-tamparan-gadis&cHash=bdc1f35f49ac6e3c2908d5a2d481d678. Accessed 17 March 2022.

———. 2008. PI.ÚS 1/08. https://www.usoud.cz/en/decisions/20080923-pl-us-108-stabilization-of-public-budget-health-care-fees-1. Accessed 17 March 2022.

———. 2013. Pl.ÚS 36/11. https://www.usoud.cz/en/decisions/20130620-pl-us-3611-standard-and-above-standard-health-care/. Accessed 17 March 2022.

ČTK. 1989a. *Rozhovor s ministrem zdravotnictví a sociálních věcí ČSR* [Interview with the Minister of Health and Social Affairs of the Czech Socialist Republic]. *Infobanka ČTK* 8 (8). http://www.ctk.cz/infobanka. Accessed 10 March 2022.

———. 1989b. *TB s ministry J.Prokopcem a A. Molnárem* [TB with ministers J. Prokopec and A. Molnár]. *Infobanka ČTK* 23 (10). http://www.ctk.cz/infobanka. Accessed 10 March 2022.

———. 1995a. *Rubáš přiznal, že na počátku měla být jedna zdravotní pojišťovna* [Rubáš admitted that there should have been one health insurance company in the beginning]. *Infobanka ČTK* 19 (5). http://www.ctk.cz/infobanka. Accessed 20 March 2022.

———. 1995b. *Buzková: Zákon o zdravotních pojišťovnách zakotví monopol VZP* [Buzková: The Act on Health Insurance Companies will entrench the VZP monopoly]. *Infobanka ČTK* 13 (3). http://www.ctk.cz/infobanka. Accessed 20 March 2022.

———. 1995c. *Přímé platby v ordinaci ne dříve než v roce 1997* [Direct payments in the doctor's office no earlier than 1997]. *Infobanka ČTK* 12 (1). http://www.ctk.cz/infobanka. Accessed 20 March 2022.

———. 1996. *Horák: Zdravotníci chtějí odměnu, která je bude motivovat* [Horák: Health workers want a reward that will motivate them] *Infobanka ČTK* 25 (3). http://www.ctk.cz/infobanka. Accessed 20 March 2022.

———. 2005. *Klaus vetoval zákon zakazující převody nemocnic* [Klaus vetoed the law prohibiting hospital transfers]. *Infobanka ČTK* 12 (9). http://www.ctk.cz/infobanka. Accessed 20 March 2022.

———. 2010. *Proplácení zdravotnických poplatků je diskriminační, míní Brusel* [Reimbursement of medical fees is discriminatory, according to Brussels]. *Infobanka ČTK* 1 (6). http://www.ctk.cz/infobanka. Accessed 20 March 2022.

Czech National Council. 1988. Resolution No. 67, 12th meeting of the Czech National Council, 1 November 1988. https://www.psp.cz/eknih/1986cnr/usneseni/u0067.htm. Accessed 10 March 2022.

Domas, Josef. 1988. Speech at the 13th meeting of the Czech National Council, 20 December 1988. https://www.psp.cz/eknih/1986cnr/stenprot/013schuz/s013011.htm. Accessed 10 March 2022.

Dvořáková, Vladimíra. 2003. Civil society in the Czech Republic: 'Impulse 99'and 'thank you, time to go'. In *Uncivil society? Contentious politics in post-communist Europe*, ed. P. Kopecky and C. Mudde, 134–156. London: Routledge.

Field, Mark G. 1991. The hybrid profession: Soviet medicine. In *Professions and the state: Expertise and autonomy in the Soviet Union and Eastern Europe*, ed. Anthony Jones. Philadelphia: Temple University.

Gibbons, Brian. 1993. Salaried general practice in Czechoslovakia: Personal observations and impressions. *British Journal of General Practice* 43 (373): 345–347.

Hanley, Seán. 2012. Dynamics of new party formation in the Czech Republic 1996–2010: Looking for the origins of a 'political earthquake'. *East European Politics* 28 (2): 119–143.

Hanley, Seán, and Milada Anna Vachudova. 2018. Understanding the illiberal turn: Democratic backsliding in the Czech Republic. *East European Politics* 34 (3): 276–296.

Háva, Petr, and Ladislav Kružík. 1995. Prùbìh privatizace v českém zdravotnictví. In *Analýza událostí veřejné politiky v České republice*, ed. M. Potůček, M. Purkrábek, and P. Háva, 54–76. Praha: Fakulta sociálních věd University Karlovy.

Havlík, Vlastimil. 2015. Stable or not? Patterns of party system dynamics and the rise of the new political parties in the Czech Republic. Romanian Journal of Political Sciences 15(1): 185–207.

Hroboň, Pavel, Tomáš Macháček, and Tomáš Julínek. 2005. *Reforma zdravotnictví pro Českou Republiku v Evropě 21*. Prague: Století.

IDNES. 2009. *Vrchní soud podpořil zákaz Rathových kliček s poplatky* [High Court upholds ban on Rath's fee loops]. https://www.idnes.cz/zpravy/domaci/vrchni-soud-podporil-zakaz-rathovych-klicek-s-poplatky.A090917_143415_domaci_taj. Accessed 17 March 2022.

———. 2010a. *Poplatky u lékaře do voleb nepadnou. ČSSD teď bitvu o ně prohrála* [Doctor's fees do not fall into the election. ČSSD has now lost the battle for them]. https://www.idnes.cz/zpravy/domaci/poplatky-u-lekare-do-voleb-nepadnou-cssd-ted-bitvu-o-ne-prohrala.A100316_172300_domaci_kop. Accessed 17 March 2022.

———. 2010b. *Před volbami se přiostřuje boj o poplatky, k soudu míří dvě ústavní stížnosti* [Before the elections, the fight over fees is intensifying, two constitutional complaints are heading to court]. https://www.idnes.cz/zpravy/domaci/pred-volbami-sili-boj-o-poplatky-k-soudu-miri-hned-dve-ustavni-stiznosti.A100205_140636_domaci_kop. Accessed 17 March 2022.

Inglot, Tomasz. 2008. *Welfare states in East Central Europe*. Cambridge: Cambridge University Press.

Jaroš, Jan, and Kamil Kalina. 1998. Czech health care system: Delivery and financing. Czech Association for Health Service Research.

Jaroš, Jan, Kamil Kalina, Martin Dlouhý, and Antonín Malina. 2005. Decentralization and governance of healthcare in the Czech Republic in the 1990s. In *Decentralization in healthcare: Analyses and experiences in Central and Eastern Europe in the 1990s*, ed. George Shakarishvili. Budapest: Local Government and Public Service Reform Initiative, Open Society Institute.

Käser, Michael. 1976. *Health care in the Soviet Union and Eastern Europe*. London: Croom Helm.

Keefer, Philip, and Mary Shirley. 2001. Privatization in transition economies: Politics as usual? In *Presidents, parliaments, and policy*, ed. S. Haggard and M.D. McCubbins, 291–319. Cambridge: Cambridge University Press.

Kitschelt, Herbert, Zdenka Mansfeldová, Radoslav Markowski, and Gábor Tóka. 1999. *Post-communist party systems: Competition, representation, and inter-party cooperation*. Cambridge: Cambridge University Press.

Klaus, Václav. 2018. Conference P. T. Bauer: A Hungarian in Cambridge, Danube Institute, Hungarian National Bank, Budapest, March 27, 2018. *Hungarian Review* 9 (3).

Kopeček, Lubomír, and Pavel Pšeja. 2008. Czech Social Democracy and its 'cohabitation' with the Communist Party: The story of a neglected affair. *Communist and Post-Communist Studies* 41 (3): 317–338.

Kopecký, Petr. 2007. Political parties in the Czech and Slovak Republics. In *Party politics in new democracies*, ed. Paul Webb and Stephen White, 119–146. Oxford: Oxford University Press.

Korbel, Josef. 1977. Twentieth-century Czechoslovakia: the meanings of its history. New York: Columbia University Press.

Langer, Ivan. 2002. Parliamentary speech by Ivan Langer. https://www.psp.cz/eknih/2002ps/stenprot/053schuz/s053373.htm#r4. Accessed 10 March 2022.

Mansfeldová, Zdenka. 2013. The Czech Republic. In *The handbook of political change in Eastern Europe*, ed. S. Berglund, J. Ekman, K. Deegan-Krause, and T. Knutsen, 339–368. Cheltenham: Edward Elgar Publishing.

Marrée, Jörgen, and Peter P. Groenewegen. 1997. *Back to Bismarck: Eastern Europe health care systems in transition*. Avebury: Ashgate.

Mihalco, Zdenek. 2007. *Kraje urychleně mění status nemocnic* [Regions are rapidly changing the status of hospitals]. https://zpravy.aktualne.cz/domaci/kraje-urychlene-meni-status-nemocnic/r~i:article:352670/. Accessed 20 March 2022.

Ministry of Health. 1990a. *Návrh reformy zdravotnictví* [Health care reform proposal]. Working Group for Reform, Ministry of Health of the Czech Republic.

———. 1990b. *Návrh nového systému zdravotní péče* [Proposal for a new health care system]. Ministry of Health of the Czech Republic.

———. 1995a. *Dlouhodobý program Ministerstva zdravotnictví* [Long-term program of the Ministry of Health]. Ministry of Health of the Czech Republic.

———. 1995b. *Krátkodobý program Ministerstva zdravotnictví* [Long-term program of the Ministry of Health]. Ministry of Health of the Czech Republic.

OECD. 2020. Healthcare resources. OECD Health Statistics (database). https://doi.org/10.1787/data-00541-en. Accessed 25 March 2022.

Potůček, Martin. 1999. *Not only the market*. Budapest: Central European University Press.

Popic, Tamara. 2021. The Czech Republic. In Health politics in Europe: A handbook, ed. E.M. Immergut, K.M. Anderson, C. Devitt, and T. Popic, 275–306. Oxford: Oxford University Press

Raffel, Marshall W., and Norma K. Raffel. 1992. Czechoslovakia's changing health care system. *Public Health Reports* 107 (6): 636–643.

Rath, David. 2006. Parliamentary speech by David Rath. https://www.psp.cz/eknih/2006ps/stenprot/018schuz/s018040.htm. Accessed 10 March 2022.

Scheffler, Richard. 1999. Lessons learned from the reform of the Czech health care system. *Česká společnost na konci tisíciletí* 2.

Stark, David, and Laszlo Bruszt. 1998. *Postsocialist pathways: Transforming politics and property in East Central Europe*. Cambridge: Cambridge University Press.

Svobodný, Petr, Helena Hnilicová, Hana Janecková, Eva Krížová, and Hana Mášová. 2004. Continuity and discontinuity of health and health care in the Czech lands during two centuries (1800–2000). *Hygiea Internationalis* 4 (1): 81–107.

van Ginneken, Ewout, Alena Ottichova, and Matthew Gaskins. 2010. User fees in the Czech Republic: The continuing story of a divisive tool. *Eurohealth* 16 (3): 1.

Vepřek, Jaromír, Pavel Vepřek, and Jaroslav Janda. 2002. *Zpráva o léčení českého zdravotnictví, aneb, Zdravotnická reforma včera, dnes a zítra*. Prague: Grada.

Weinerman, E. Richard. 1969. *Social medicine in Eastern Europe: The organization of health services and the education of medical personnel in Czechoslovakia, Hungary, and Poland*. Cambridge: Harvard University Press.

World Bank. 1991. *The Czech and Slovak federal republic: Issues and priorities in the healthcare sector*. Washington, DC: Europe and Central Asia, Middle East and North Africa Regions, Human Resource Operation Division.

CHAPTER 5

Poland

Introduction

This chapter accounts for the origins and main developments of the Polish post-communist health reforms. Its elaborate empirical analysis explains why policymakers' efforts to introduce different types of markets in the health system had limited success, and the policy learning process was marked by reversals and failures. The chapter tracks the origins of market reforms in the socialist period, showing how anomalies in the Soviet-style policy paradigm generated an ideational shift indicated by a departure from the state-led healthcare model based on hierarchical resource distribution and central planning. Like the Czech health policymakers in early post-socialism, the Polish policymakers relied on the new market ideas and opted for a radical approach to reform. They resisted the influence of foreign experts but faced a series of implementation failures. In contrast to the Czech and Slovenian cases, because of stronger party divisionsmarked by sharp political conflicts, and thick veto configurations, the Polish health policy witnessed a series of reversals that not only re-introduced a state-dominated monopsony in healthcare financing, but also prevented further marketisation attempts.

Similar to the Slovenian case, however, the Polish case is curious from a theoretical point of view. Given the constitutionally defined thick veto configurations, we might assume strong institutional constraints on the policy process and therefore expect a lack of policy change. Yet, the Polish

T. Popic, *Health Reforms in Post-Communist Eastern Europe*,
https://doi.org/10.1007/978-3-031-15497-3_5

health policy took a dramatic U-turn in the early 2000s. This points to the limits of explanations of policy change focusing exclusively on institutional vetoes and underlines the importance of party politics (see Popic 2021a). As shown in this chapter, when parties' dynamics include strong divisions over certain healthcare issues, and the political arrangements absorb constitutionally established vetoes, the result can be a major policy reshuffling in spite of thick institutional constraints.

The chapter proceeds as follows. The first part explains Polish healthcare under socialism, showing how after the successful implementation of the Soviet-style healthcare system, a series of anomalies led to the decline of the socialist policy paradigm and the emergence of market-oriented ideas. The next part analyses key policy episodes from the post-communist period: the privatisation of primary care, the shift to a decentralised, competitive insurance system and its reversal, and attempts to privatise public hospitals. The final section summarises the main developments in the country's post-communist health policy, marked by policy *reversals*, in contrast to Slovenian *survival* and Czech *instability*.

Polish Healthcare Under Socialism

In the early post-war period, Poland established the Soviet-style 'Semashko' healthcare system. This included the nationalisation of healthcare facilities and the introduction of a centralised model of healthcare provision based on socialist planning that gradually led to universal coverage. Despite the considerable success of the socialist system in providing healthcare for all, anomalies became evident in population health outcomes, leading to crisis and generating discussions of possible solutions. Whilst the solutions of the socialist regime were ineffective, the crisis of the socialist healthcare paradigm set the stage for the post-communist health policy debate, triggering policy change and sparking a turbulent learning process.

Introduction of the Socialist Policy Paradigm

The Soviet liberation of Poland, followed by the occupation and the first post-war elections in 1947 and rise to power of the communist party, the Polish United Worker's Party (*Polska Zjednoczona Partia Robotnicza—PZPR*), in 1948, led to the establishment of socialism through an official proclamation of the People's Republic of Poland. During the pre-war period, the country's healthcare system was based on the insurance model, and the shift to the Semashko system took place during the first post-war years.[1] A series of laws passed in the 1940s and 1950s as amendments to the 1933 Law on Social Insurance created a national health service system with a centralised administration (Popic 2021b: 748).[2]

Subsequent changes included the establishment of the Ministry of Health and Social Welfare in 1945; healthcare facilities became ministerial responsibilities, that is, placed under the direct control of the central state. Another post-war change was the replacement of health insurance contributions previously shared equally by employers and employees with a system of contributions paid solely by employers. The final steps in the implementation of the Semashko model involved two changes in 1951. One was the incorporation of the sickness funds into the general budget and the shift of healthcare financing from contributions to general taxation, and the other was the abolition of the Polish Chamber of Physicians and regional professional medical associations (Roemer and Roemer 1981).

Universal and free healthcare was an important element in the post-war political programme of the socialist regime, seen as a tool for establishing equity in health status. Thus, the 1952 Constitution introduced the universal right to healthcare. The elimination of financial barriers to medical goods and services aimed to intensify the use of these resources by the underprivileged social classes and therefore served as legitimation of the new regime (Włodarczyk 1987). As a universal health system required a larger professional medical workforce, significant attention during the post-war restructuring was given to education of medical personnel. By 1950, the proportion of doctors had reached the pre-war level of 3.7 per 10,000 inhabitants, rising to 6.7 by 1955 (Millard 1982). The endorsement of Soviet-style socialised medicine also included the establishment of occupational health clinics in workplaces across the country.

Polish healthcare under socialism mirrored the Soviet-style healthcare systems across the Eastern Bloc, but it had a unique feature: private healthcare services were not formally abolished (Karski et al. 1999). This meant some doctors and dentists continued offering their services through private medical cooperatives throughout the socialist period. However, rather

[1] During the inter-war period, Polish healthcare was based on an insurance system similar to German, that is, Bismarckian system of sickness funds with a territorial structure (Popic 2021b).

[2] 1944, 1946, 1947, 1948, 1951, and 1954 Amendments to the Law on Social Insurance (*Ustawa o ubezpieczeniu społecnem*).

than showing the openness of the socialist regime to the integration of market elements, the private provision was a remnant of the past and was left in place to ensure population groups not covered by the state system, mainly Polish farmers, could have access to healthcare (Popic 2021b).

In the first decades following World War II, Poland saw significant progress in healthcare coverage and provision, evident in the improved health status of the population. In the 1950s and early 1960s, mainly due to mandatory immunisation and compulsory programmes of medical treatment, the country eliminated many infectious diseases, and some of the main indicators of population health, such as life expectancy and infant mortality, improved dramatically (Golinowska and Sowa 2006).

The Socialist Health Crisis

The first signs that this 'golden age' of the Polish socialist healthcare might be over appeared in the mid-1960s. Anomalies became evident in the worsening of the health status, in particular, an increase in men's mortality rates (Golinowska and Sowa 2006). In the day-to-day provision of medical services, anomalies appeared because of constant underfunding. The introduction of the Soviet-style Stalinist model of socio-economic organisation in the post-war period meant priority in spending was given to heavy industry; health and other social services were considered 'non-productive sectors' and remained underfinanced (Pieprzyk 2013).

Another sector-related problem was the vertical fragmentation of service delivery. Even though most health facilities were controlled by the Ministry of Health, individual hospitals, separate emergency services, outpatient clinics, and occupational health clinics functioned as autonomous units without horizontal links (Millard 1982). This meant the delivery of services was divided into separate vertical structures; this hindered coordination and fostered inefficient use of resources, low productivity and inadequate supervision and control. The system also showed elements of dysfunctionality because of the tendency to focus on specialised care. The primacy of specialised care undermined the work of generalist physicians and increased the workload of specialists; this, in turn, contributed to low morale amongst healthcare professionals and, in combination with underfunding, was seen as leading to corruption (Millard 1982; Włodarczyk 1987).

Deficiencies of the Polish health sector stimulated discussion on ways out of the crisis. In the late 1960s, a commission of experts from the Union of Healthcare Service Workers developed a proposal for healthcare reform. The proposal pointed to the organisational fragmentation of the system and existing methods of financing as two root causes of inefficiency in service provision. It suggested reform focused mainly on organisational change and envisaged a system of integrated healthcare. This system would establish a single organisational unit at the county level to provide primary, dental, and emergency care, as well as a limited range of specialist services, through outpatient clinics and a general hospital (Millard 1982).

The problems of the healthcare sector were noted by the socialist establishment as well. Its openness to discussions about health and the broader socio-economic crisis was partially due to a leadership change in the Polish Communist Party—the 1970 rise of reformer Edward Gierek. In an attempt to solve the healthcare problems, Gierek announced a series of reforms at the Sixth Party Congress in December 1971, presenting a long-term strategy of socio-economic development and designated healthcare as the area of highest priority (Millard 1982; Inglot 2008).

The new regime's strategy included two key changes. One was the immediate expansion of healthcare coverage to farmers,[3] a large population hitherto lacking access to the public healthcare system (Roemer and Roemer 1981). The other was the re-organisation of healthcare delivery through the introduction of integrated Healthcare Units (*Zespół Opieki Zdrawotnej—ZOZ*). The establishment of ZOZs was based on the previous reform proposal of the Union of Healthcare Service Workers and was integrated into the government's long-term plan, 'Programme for the Development of Healthcare and Social Welfare until 1990', presented to Parliament in 1973.[4] This programme envisaged nationwide introduction of ZOZs; the plan was to integrate services of primary care, hospital, emergency and specialist care, and even welfare assistance locally, at the county level (Kuszewski et al. 2005). From a political perspective, the introduction of this programme represented Gierek's attempt to convince Polish society of the government's commitment to healthcare improvement (Millard 1982).

Yet, the problems of Polish healthcare remained unsolved. The healthcare sector continued to be underfunded, experiencing shortages of staff, equipment, and basic supplies, all of which diminished the potentially

[3] Rozporządzenie Ministra Zdrowia i Opieki Społecznej z 14 grudnia 1971 r. w sprawie udzielania świadczeń leczniczych przez zakłady społeczne służby zdrowia osobom prowadzącym gospodarstwa rolne.

[4] Program Rozwoju Ochrony Zdrowia i Opieki Społecznej do 1990.

beneficial effects of the organisational integration (Millard 1982). More importantly, the introduction of ZOZs was not perceived as systemic change; in fact, these new management units were seen as evidence of further bureaucratisation (Włodarczyk 1987; Włodarczyk and Karkowska 2000). The failure of the ZOZs to solve the healthcare problems also reflected the more general failure of Gierek's vision of state socialism—in effect, it promised more than it could deliver (Inglot 2008: 166).

During the late 1970s, the worsening of healthcare was noted and criticised by the public and the press (Millard 1982). These criticisms were followed by a renewed discussion of the healthcare system's future at the Central Committee of the Communist Party in June 1980 (Włodarczyk 1987). During this discussion, held at a special plenary session of the Committee dedicated exclusively to the problems of the health sector, Minister of Health Marian Słiwinski confessed that despite considerable effort, there was a lack of progress (Słiwinski 1980). Shortly after this confession, Słiwinski resigned from his ministerial position.

Political reshuffling also involved change in the Party leadership, as Stanisłav Kania was replaced in 1981 by General Wojciech Jaruzelski. The Jaruzelski regime introduced Martial Law in 1981 and issued the Parliamentary Resolution on Health Care and Social Welfare in 1983. This Resolution evaluated the health status of the Polish population as satisfactory and declared that, despite the extremely difficult economic situation, the healthcare sector was performing well (Sejm 1983).

Emergence of Market Ideas

During the last decade of socialist rule, despite the broad socio-economic reforms under Jaruzelski's leadership, the Polish healthcare system remained relatively unchanged. The only changes were the introduction of a small degree of flexibility in healthcare organisation and the free choice of physicians in a very limited number of urban health centres (Włodarczyk 1987). The 1980s were also characterised by efforts to strengthen the administrative powers of provinces and municipalities (Karski et al. 1999). Even though these changes were not dramatic, they had symbolic importance because they went against the extremely rigid control-and-command logic of the centralised model of socialist healthcare management.

Yet, the absence of systemic change by the late 1980s implied the constant underfunding, shortages, low salaries, and high levels of corruption had become ubiquitous characteristics of the Polish healthcare sector. Corruption in particular became so rooted that it was a regular element of both individual healthcare expenditures and physicians' incomes (Tymowska 1987).[5] The dysfunctionality of the system was continuously reflected in the worsening of the population health, including reductions in life expectancy and drastically increased rates of deaths caused by non-communicable diseases (Marrée and Groenewegen 1997: 100).

The deepening crisis of health and healthcare prompted the emergence of new ideas questioning the core of the socialist health paradigm. The first open criticism of the key tenets of the socialist health system was published in the early 1980s as part of a bigger report written by a group of experts associated with the anti-regime trade union Solidarity (*Solidarność*).[6] This report diagnosed the healthcare system as substantially underfunded, chronically lacking medicines, and experiencing constant shortages of medical equipment and materials, all of which generated tragic situations in Polish hospitals. The report claimed that due to the lack of resources, it had become impossible for the system to meet the existing health needs. Looking more broadly, the report suggested the deficiencies of the health sector were systemic, a consequence of poor system management which was completely ineffective and not able to rationally distribute healthcare resources.

Other expert reports on healthcare issues appeared during the 1980s suggesting more concrete policy changes. One report, for example, advised regionalisation and greater flexibility in the organisational structure of the healthcare system. It argued the main source of the systemic problems was the evaluation of managerial performance on the basis of rigid and ineffective criteria and suggested these should be replaced by the criterion of efficiency.[7] Another report went even further, proposing the (re)introduction of an insurance system coupled with a definition of a basic package of healthcare services.[8] Whilst services in this package would be covered by the public health system, those outside the package, such as

[5] It is difficult to estimate the degree of healthcare corruption under socialism, but Tymowska (1987) estimated 0.5 per cent of GDP should be added to the official records of the total healthcare spending to account for the scope of the informal payments.

[6] *Raport Konwersatorium 'Doświaczeienie i Przyszłość', Zycie i Nowoczesność*, 02 April 1981.

[7] Interview No. 20.

[8] Dawydzik L, Gdulewicz T, Indulski J, Smoleń M, Włodarczyk C, Wysocki J. Directions of health system reform. Warsaw, December 1988–January 1989.

services offering more sophisticated care, would be paid by voluntary health insurance (Smoleń 1992).

The publication of critical reports pressed the socialist leadership to seek solutions for the sector's problems, especially in the context of increasing political pressures generated by frequent strikes organised by Solidarity. In 1988, the Ministry of Health published a High Commission Report, 'Draft Reform of the Health and Social Care'. Based on the commissioned opinion of a group of healthcare experts, this report was the first official document openly calling for the replacement of the existing budget-based system with an insurance system of healthcare financing. According to this report, the shift to the insurance system would increase desperately needed financial resources through insurance contributions; even more importantly, it would establish a more rational model for resource distribution. It would also supply a new set of incentives in which the insurance funds would pay healthcare providers not on the basis of a previously established budget but according to the services they actually provided, that is, according to their performance (Ministry of Health and Social Care 1988).

The experts' report and the Ministry's reform document suggested a vibrant dynamic within Polish healthcare policy circles—a cognitive break with the socialist paradigm and a turn towards market-oriented ideas. However, these ideas were shelved in the context of the heated political conflict between the Jaruzelski regime and the anti-regime forces represented by Solidarity; this ultimately resulted in the Round Table Talks and Agreement in autumn 1989.

Institutional and Political Context of Post-Communist Health Reform

The Polish healthcare policy in the 1980s can be characterised as a period of very interesting and stimulating reform ideas, but also as a period of 'extreme scarcity of decisions' (Indulski and Włodarczyk 1989: 19). In spite of the vibrant policy debate under late socialism, Poland remained faithful to the socialist paradigm of the state-dominated, command-and-control system of healthcare until the regime change in 1989. Nevertheless, the ideas about healthcare reform put forward in late socialism were fundamental for the post-communist reforms in two main respects. One was that they formulated the 'diagnosis', that is, views on the source of problems in the country's healthcare system; these were characterised as systemic problems of the socialist healthcare. By pointing to underfunding and shortages and finding the causes of these problems in the rigidity of the existing system, they suggested the real cause of the problem was the incapacity of the system to manage resources. The other was that these ideas offered a 'cure' for the diagnosed problems, blueprints for reform, suggesting a market-oriented insurance system with a different set of incentives and modes of healthcare provision would be a way out of the crisis.

Yet, in the post-communist period, the translation of these market ideas into policy turned out to be a rather difficult task. The lack of policy legacies that involved experience with markets in healthcare had a crucial impact on the initial health policy choices, leading Polish reformers to opt for more radical reform options that generated implementation failures and resulted in a return to a centralised system. Moreover, the combination of an institutional setup of thick veto configurations and a strong political conflict over health issues meant the subsequent reform process was uneven, featuring continuous attempts at marketisation fraught with failure.

Institutions: Thick Veto Points Configuration

Waves of anti-regime strikes organised by Solidarity forced Jaruzelski's government to start negotiating regime transition with the opposition through a series of Round Table Talks in 1989. With the government and the Solidarity leaders as the main participants, these Talks resulted in a regime-opposition compromise whereby transition from the communist to a democratic system would be handled gradually (Elster 1996; Stark and Bruszt 1998). The unique character of the Polish compromise-based extrication from communism had a strong influence on the country's new constitutional architecture.

With the gradual shift to a fully democratic system and on-going political conflicts between the communists and anti-communists, the new Constitution was passed only in 1997. Formally proclaimed by the government led by the communist successor party Democratic Left Alliance (*Sojusz Lewicy Demokratycznej*—SLD), the Constitution established Poland as a parliamentary democracy with a strong element of semi-presidentialism (Pelczynski and Kowalski 1990; McMenamin 2008).

The country's bi-cameral Parliament represented one of the main veto point arenas with conditional veto powers; the decisions made by the Sejm as the Parliament's Lower House could be vetoed by the Senate as its Upper House, but the Sejm was still able to overrule this veto by the absolute majority of its votes (Constitution of the Republic of Poland 1997, Art. 121). In addition, the Constitution gave strong veto powers to the President as the Head of state. It specified the Parliament's decisions could be vetoed by the President, but defined this veto as conditional, stipulating it could be overruled by the Sejm with three fifths of its votes (Constitution of the Republic of Poland 1997, Art. 122). The higher share of the Sejm's votes required to overturn the President's (three fifths, i.e., 60 per cent) than the Senate's veto (50 per cent) meant the President had strong prerogatives in the policymaking process.[9] As the Constitutional Court was also given the right to make checks on constitutionality initiated by the public, it was provided with veto powers in the judicial arena. The electorate was the last veto point arena, with the power to overthrow or accept government's decisions through a referendum.

This new institutional architecture became crucial for Poland's health policy and its trajectories throughout the post-communist period. The institutional setup of bicameralism, semi-presidentialism, and veto powers of the Constitutional Court and the electorate generated a system of checks and balances featuring a relatively thick veto points' structure (see Chap. 2). As this chapter goes on to show, this thick institutional structure, combined with fierce party competition over health policy, played a decisive role in the policymaking process, generating a series of policy deadlocks and reversals over three decades.

Party Politics: Strong Party Divisions on Health Policy

As mentioned earlier, Poland's extrication from state socialism was marked by 'compromise', the result of the Round Table negotiations between the leaders of the communist regime and Solidarity (Stark and Bruszt 1998). During the negotiations, the position of the Polish communist party was still strong, so Solidarity made a pragmatic compromise, agreeing to give the presidency to the communist party, but receiving in return the

[9] Until 1997, the Lower House needed two-thirds (66.66 per cent) of votes to overturn the veto; thus, the 1997 provisions weakened the presidential veto (Popic 2021b).

leadership of the government. Another core result of the negotiations was that the election of the Sejm was organised on a unique system of 'compartmentalised competition': only part of the parliamentary seats were open for electoral competition; the rest were reserved for the communist party (Olson 1993).[10] This compromise reached at the Round Table did not match the expectations of the Solidarity leaders, as the communist party was guaranteed partial but nevertheless continued control of the country's main political institutions, without being exposed to the uncertainties of electoral competition.

Even though the shift to a free and competitive system took place in the 1990 presidential and the 1991 parliamentary elections, the 1990s and early 2000s were politically turbulent. Conflict between the new, post-Solidarity parties and the communist successor parties resulted in political instability, with frequent government changes in the context of a highly under-institutionalised party system. In the first fully competitive election, Solidarity split into pieces, with 29 post-Solidarity groups entering Parliament (Millard 2009). Over time, however, these groups managed to unite into a large post-Solidarity political formation, Solidarity Election Action (*Akcja Wyborcza Solidarność—AWS*). This electoral alliance brought together more than 33 centre-right parties in 1996 (Szczerbiak 2002). The AWS won the election in 1997, and formed a government in coalition with another post-Solidarity party, Freedom Union (*Unia Wolności—UW*).

In terms of broader socio-economic reforms, the post-Solidarity parties were responsible for Poland's 'shock therapy', stressing rapid transformation into capitalism in the form of radical macroeconomic reforms, justified by the fear of the possible return of the communist regime. The therapy, led by the country's first post-communist Prime Minister, Leszek Balcerowitz, and hence also called the 'Balcerowitz Plan', featured a series of measures including, among other, reducing wages in the public sector, eliminating subsidies and price controls, and privatising previously public enterprises.

Given the focus on economic restructuring, the first post-Solidarity government led by Tadeusz Mazowiecki (1991–1993) was conservative in pursuing welfare reform, focusing on continuity and leaving the Poland's social policy largely unreformed (see Inglot 2008: 255). Unfortunately,

[10] Sixty-five per cent of the seats in the Sejm were reserved for the communist party and its satellites, and 35 per cent were open for competition (Olson 1993).

the 'shock therapy' triggered a dramatic decline in the country's economy; this was coupled with a jump in inflation and unemployment, thus further slowing welfare reform. The economic context was exacerbated by disagreements amongst the post-Solidarity parties (see Guardiancich 2012). Despite internal strife, Jerzy Buzek's AWS-UW government, established in 1997, finally managed to introduce large-scale welfare reforms, including a shift to an insurance based healthcare system

The main political opponent of the post-Solidarity political parties was the communist successor party—the Democratic Left Alliance (SLD). Like the AWS, the SLD comprised a number of trade unions and social organisations that had enjoyed patronage during the communist period, but it was dominated by the Social Democracy of the Republic of Poland party (*Socjaldemokracja Rzeczpospolitej Polskiej—SdRP*), formed as a successor to the Polish United Workers Party (Szczerbiak 2002).[11] In sharp contrast to the most of the communist successor parties in the Eastern Bloc, the SLD had electoral success very early, winning the largest portion of votes in the 1993 elections. Poles' decision to bring the communists back into power so quickly after the Round Table Talks was seen as a response to the radical economic reforms pushed by Solidarity at the start of the transition (Ekiert and Kubik 2001). SLD's success and its presence in Polish transitional politics was confirmed by the victory of the party's founder, Aleksander Kwaśniewski, in the 1995 presidential elections.[12] This early and huge electoral success made the SLD strong and assertive; even though the party lost to the AWS in 1997, its massive victory in the 2001 election confirmed party's hegemony on the Polish left (Millard 2009).

In the context of the debate over the first major health reform, the introduction of the insurance system, the SLD opposed the radical neoliberal solutions proposed by the post-Solidarity forces, but showed a willingness to negotiate and accept reforms allowing for some elements of markets in the new system. This position can be explained by an important aspect of the political context of the early transition—the SLD's identity change and transformation into a flexible party of social democratic orientation (Grzymała-Busse 2002; Millard 2006). As a communist successor party, the SLD saw its legitimacy partly conditional on continuing the policies of the post-Solidarity period, assuring voters that the reforms they

[11] Until 2000, SLD's name was Social Democracy of the Republic of Poland (*Socjaldemokracja Rzeczypospolitej Polskiej—SdRP*).

[12] Kwaśniewski was the leader of Social Democracy (*SdRP*).

were willing to support were in line with the Third Way; they reflected liberal social democratic ideas, not the strong anti-market, statist ideas of central government control (see c and Włodarczyk 2000). Yet, the inter-party conflict over health reform sharpened after series of failures in the implementation of the new insurance system, especially as this generated large public discontent. In the 2001 elections, the SLD adroitly and opportunistically shifted the blame for failed reforms to the AWS and included a new round of health reform in its electoral promises (Krajewski-Siuda and Romaniuk 2008).

However, SLD's new health reform, including re-centralisation of the insurance system, was highly controversial and was followed by a major reshuffling of the country's political landscape after the 2005 elections. The electoral demise of the left generated a yet another round of reform dynamics shaped by the two right-wing parties, the conservative Law and Justice (PiS) and the liberal Civic Platform (PO). Even though in the more general socio-economic programmes, the two parties showed a willingness to collaborate, their position on some of the core healthcare reforms such as hospital privatisation remained sharply divided. The rivalry between the PiS and PO was fuelled by the victory of PiS leader Lech Kaczyński in the 2005 presidential elections, when he defeated PO leader Donald Tusk (see McMenamin 2008). Kaczyński was one of the most vocal opponents of the PO's plans for hospital reforms, and already in the first months of Kaczyński's presidency, the rivalry between the two parties was heightened. The party conflict peaked in 2008 when Kaczyński vetoed plans for commercialisation of public hospitals, which envisaged their transformation into joint-stock companies. From a theoretical perspective, this policy episode demonstrated that whether and to what extent ideas can influence policy depends not only on the institutional structures of political power that could potentially constrain the policy process, but also on the context of party competition (see Chap. 2).

Key Episodes in Post-Communist Healthcare Reform

Initial Post-Communist Reform Debate

Healthcare reforms were discussed during the Round Table Talks, with one of the sessions specifically dedicated to the topic. The basis for the discussion was a proposal published in the late 1980s, co-authored by a group of experts, suggesting the introduction of a basic benefit package and an insurance system combined with a private, voluntary element. The insurance system was included in the Round Table Agreement, but the idea of a basic package combined with voluntary insurance for 'extra' services was angrily rejected by the communists (Smoleń 1992).

The first, semi-free elections took place in June 1989 with Solidarity winning all but one seat in the Sejm, and the government was formed under Tadeusz Mazowiecki. Two competing draft proposals for healthcare reform were developed under Mazowiecki's government. 'Proposal for Reform' was developed by a Solidarity-based group of healthcare experts positioned within the Committee for Reforms in Healthcare and Social Welfare Systems in the Ministry of Health (Włodarczyk and Mierzewski 1991). This expert group took control of the policy design because the Minister had not articulated a position on healthcare.[13] The group argued the Round Table Agreement should become the Ministry's official proposal for reform (Ministry of Health and Social Care 1988). The proposal included the creation of a central, independent health insurance fund with separate branches, funded by employers' contributions and public funds, and it suggested the consideration of private forms of ownership of healthcare facilities. It also suggested a shift from the reimbursement for services based on a pre-established budget to a new method of reimbursement based on types and quantities of services (Smoleń 1992; Bossert and Włodarczyk 2000).

Simultaneously, a competing proposal emerged. 'In the Interest of the Health of Society' was prepared by an independent team of experts outside the Ministry and therefore was also called the 'Independent Proposal' (Golinowska et al. 1989).[14] Similar to the Ministry's proposal, this one envisioned a central healthcare insurance fund, but took a stronger state-oriented stance, arguing the health insurance fund should be dependent on the Ministry of Health and insisting on public provision of healthcare services. It also argued the insurance contributions should be paid by both employers and employees, and the insurance fund should be partially financed by the state budget. Rather than reimbursement for services by type or quantity, healthcare providers would be paid on the basis of ex-ante global budgets, and these would cover all expenses in the coming year (Bossert and Włodarczyk 2000).

[13] Interview No. 20.

[14] Interview No. 29.

The differences between the first two post-communist proposals for health reform were illustrative of a divide over health issues that only grew bigger over time. In addition to the different views of reform, there was a considerable emotional conflict amongst the authors of the two proposals, coupled with disagreement over the exact roles of the expert groups in the reform process. The Ministry appeared to favour the 'Independent Proposal' because of its strong statist stance, but felt bound to respect the formal process of the Round Table Agreement which obliged it to support the official proposal drafted by the Ministry-based team (Bossert and Włodarczyk 2000).

The differences and disagreements generated confusion amongst the political elites (Bossert and Włodarczyk 2000), who lacked policy experience with the insurance system and were therefore unable to make decisions on the exact course of the reform. This confusion prompted the Ministry to look for help from abroad by organising a conference on health reforms with the participation of international organisations and foreign experts.[15] A conference co-sponsored by the World Health Organisation (WHO) and the World Bank (WB) resulted in a document titled 'The Political Framework of Healthcare Reform in Poland' (Ministry of Health and Social Welfare 1992). It was submitted to the Parliamentary Health Commission in March 1990 and gained formal approval (Włodarczyk and Mierzewski 1991). However, this document was soon abandoned, as the international involvement failed to bring the expert groups closer together (Bossert and Włodarczyk 2000).

Poland entered into its first recession shortly after the introduction of the transitional economic restructuring using 'shock therapy'. The worsening of the economic situation generated additional calls for health reform, but the plans to introduce an insurance system were at a standstill because of the experts' disagreement over its arrangements. The continuing conflict prompted another attempt by the Ministry of Health to seek help from international actors. This happened under the second post-communist government, led by Jan Bielecki, and the third government, led by Jan Olszewski. Olszewski replaced the members of the Ministry of Health with reform-oriented experts and political figures. In 1992, Olszewski's government started preparing a reform proposal linked to a loan agreement with the World Bank (Bossert and Włodarczyk 2000).

[15] Interview No. 20.

Consequently, the Bank's official report included recommendations for Poland's health reform (World Bank 1992).

The recommendations in the Bank's report were remarkable in that they did not follow the Bank's usual neo-liberal approach focused on markets and privatisation as solutions for welfare policy problems (see Cerami 2006). Instead, the recommendations were rather conservative, suggesting the Polish healthcare system should be focused more on improving coordination and planning within the sector than on introducing radical reforms aimed at introducing a competitive insurance system. An even more interesting aspect of the Bank report was that in marked contrast to the consensus of Polish experts, it expressed strong doubts about the shift to an insurance system. Fearing the country's instable economic outlook would make the introduction of an insurance system risky, it argued healthcare should continue to be financed by the central state budget and suggested adding new taxes, local government contributions, and co-payments as a way of improving healthcare financing. More specifically, the Bank argued:

> The budgetary system needs to be reorganized to strengthen regional resource allocation and budgeting. The ideological debate on how and from where to collect revenues continues to dominate the reform process and deflects serious attention from concrete action to improve the budgetary allocation and service delivery processes. There is no ideal Western system for Poland to copy. (World Bank 1992: xviv)

In its recommendations for healthcare delivery, the Bank's report reflected the fear of international experts that with their radical solutions, the post-communist reformers might 'throw out the baby with the bathwater' (see Barr 1994: 290). Accordingly, the Bank's experts advised the Polish reformers to keep the relatively well-functioning integrated system of healthcare provision based on the ZOZs established under socialism. The report also suggested the reformers should focus on centralised approaches to reduce the current system's inefficiencies, such as duplication of services by different providers. In terms of payments for healthcare providers, it took a statist stance, suggesting payment through budgetary transfers rather than quantity or type of care based reimbursement methods, such as capitation or fees-for-service (World Bank 1992; see also Kaminska et al. 2021).

The report of the World Bank was rejected by the government, suggesting foreign actors had little influence on the reform process in Poland (see Kaasch 2015). Defending its own views which relied on the consensus to shift to an insurance model of healthcare financing, the government argued the Bank's ideas were faulty and would not attract political support. The Polish experts, who preferred their own proposals to those of the international experts, also rejected the Bank's report. They simply argued the Bank's ideas were too similar to the old socialist system.[16] As a result, when the government signed the loan agreement with the Bank, its recommendations for health reform were ignored and quickly replaced by a new set of competing proposals under the following post-Solidarity governments.

Privatisation of Primary Care

The post-Solidarity government under Bilecki made the first step towards the integration of market-oriented elements into Polish healthcare. The ideas for privatisation of primary care were developed by a small expert team from the Ministry of Health in the form of a draft law. This draft suggested decentralisation, which would reduce the Ministry's competencies for the provision of healthcare, devolving these competencies to the level of provinces and, to a lesser extent, municipalities. Using the British Hospital Trust model for inspiration, the experts' proposal included reforms that would lead to the financial autonomy of healthcare providers, such as a purchaser–provider split. In addition, it suggested the establishment of fully independent, private healthcare providers.

The experts' ideas for changes in the provision of primary care raised no significant concerns. Whilst this might seem surprising, given the conflict over the insurance system (discussed in the next section), it can be explained by the existence of private care in Poland under communism. Initially provided for Polish farmers who were later integrated into the public system, private healthcare continued to be available until the end of the socialist period (Tymowska 1987). Making primary care private in the post-communist period was seen as allowing the easier exit of doctors from the public system and, more importantly, as giving private health provision an appropriate regulatory framework.[17] This could also explain

[16] Interview No. 20.
[17] Interview No. 28.

why during the experts' debate on the above-mentioned draft, the suggested changes were presented as purely management issues, rather than major restructuring.[18] In any event, the proposed changes were approved and passed relatively smoothly in the Sejm as the 1991 Law on Healthcare Institutions.[19]

The main changes introduced by this law were decentralisation, privatisation of healthcare facilities, and purchaser–provider split. The law eliminated the strictly unified and centralised system of healthcare facility organisation and allowed different types of facility ownership. These included ownership by central, provincial, and local authorities, but also voluntary ownership, that is, non-governmental and non-profit, and private 'for profit' arrangements.[20] The law established the legal basis for the substantial financial autonomy of publicly-owned health facilities and specified strict standards of healthcare delivery, in terms of such aspects as personnel and medical equipment (Karski et al. 1999). It also specified a comprehensive basic package of healthcare services to be offered by all types of providers, both public and private, excluding only few services such as cosmetic surgery. Finally, it introduced patient protection by granting some basic patient rights, including a right to informed consent, a right to access one's own medical records, and a right to privacy.[21]

In 1993, this law was complemented by an additional regulation of the Ministry of Health according to which the lower-level administrative units, provinces and municipalities, were allowed to enter into contracts with healthcare providers, with their own choice of reimbursement schemes.[22] Implementation of these new provisions led to gradual privatisation, mainly in primary and ambulatory care, resulting in 90 per cent of all primary care in the country becoming private by 2000 (Kuszewski et al. 2005: 90). Provinces and municipalities also experimented with different reimbursement schemes using capitation, fees per visit, fees per procedure, fees per day, or even a mix of schemes (Bossert and Włodarczyk 2000).

[18] Interview No. 20.

[19] *Ustawa o zakładach opieki zdrowotnej*, Law No. 91/408.

[20] Law No. 91/408.

[21] Law No. 91/409, Art. 19.

[22] *Rozporządzenie Ministra Zdrowia i Opieki Społecznej z dnia 5 sierpnia 1993 r. w sprawie ogólnych warunków, trybu zawierania i rozwiązywania umów o udzielanie świadczeń zdrowotnych oraz trybu ustalania i rozliczania należności za te świadczenia*] Reg. No. 76/363.

Introduction of Social Health Insurance

Whilst healthcare delivery reforms enjoyed relatively smooth sailing, healthcare financing reforms were controversial and became trapped in a protracted policy debate. The first extensive debate over the different plans for the introduction of the insurance system took place under the government of Hanna Suchocka in 1992, with four competing proposals presented for discussion (Włodarczyk and Karkowska 2000). These proposals reflected the political climate of this post-Solidarity government, which was based on a coalition of the social liberal Democratic Union (UD) and six smaller parties, including parties with Christian-democratic, conservative, and agrarian orientations, and even a beer-loving party (ZcHN, KLD, PSL-PL, PchD, and PPPP). This eclectic political mix led to disagreement, worsening conflict, and finally a policy stalemate.

The first of the four proposals was prepared by the government body responsible for the coordination of social policy, the Committee for Social Policy (Ministry of Health and Social Welfare 1992). The second was authored by an influential group of experts associated with the Solidarity trade union movement (Solidarity Trade Union 1993). The proposals were similar and were presented as a joint proposal to Parliament, suggesting introduction of an insurance system based on a large number of independent, competitive insurance funds, healthcare delivery based on predominantly private provision, and a fee-for-service reimbursement scheme. They were market-oriented and consistent with Solidarity's orientation towards privatisation and competition, but even though they clearly favoured the interests of medical professionals, they did not gain support within professional circles. For one thing, professionals found it difficult to understand how the envisaged insurance system would affect their interests. For another, there was growing conflict amongst the professional groups divided into the public and the growing private sector.[23] It took a while for the renewed Chamber of Physicians[24] and major professional associations to realise that the two proposals were in their interest and to decide to support them. The two proposals also enjoyed support of both the major part of the government and the Solidarity base of the coalition.

[23] Interview No. 21.

[24] Polish Chamber of Physicians was re-established in 1989.

The third, competing proposal was developed by an inter-ministerial team responsible for developing a broader vision of Poland's post-communist social policy reform. This team was composed of members from the Ministry of Health and Social Welfare, the Ministry of Labour, and the Ministry of Finance, all of whom belonged to Suchocka's party, the liberal Democratic Union. Instead of a competitive insurance system, this inter-ministerial team suggested a system based on regional healthcare funds combined with the public delivery of services, particularly in the hospital sector. It endorsed the existing public model of integrated care, but suggested possibilities for private provision of outpatient care (Government of Poland 1992).

The fourth proposal was developed by a team from the Government Representative Office, the part of government responsible for reform of public administration. This team was dominated by members of the Democratic Union, but this was a more liberal faction which strongly favoured decentralisation. Unsurprisingly, this team's proposal for healthcare reform was closely linked to its plan for public administration reform. This plan stipulated creation of counties (*powiats*) as new administrative units and was primarily interested in defining their role in healthcare organisation and financing. The plan did not address the health insurance issues, but it stressed the importance of public responsibility for both financing and delivery of healthcare through the county governments (Government of Poland 1993).

Two of these proposals, the joint proposal of the Social Committee and Solidarity and the proposal of the inter-ministerial team, were submitted as competing proposals to the Sejm's Health Committee. During the discussion, the inter-ministerial proposal was overwhelmingly rejected, with Committee members arguing it was not offering solutions; rather, it favoured the unacceptable status quo and, most importantly, did not reflect public expectations of the radical health reform promised in the Round Table Agreement. During the parliamentary discussion, the majority of the Sejm's members, even those from the left-wing opposition, the Polish People Party (PSL) and the SLD, supported the market-oriented proposal of the Social Committee and Solidarity, but the Democratic Union, the largest party of the governing coalition, was less enthusiastic. In the meantime, the governing coalition experienced growing political divisions because of the larger conflict between the Democratic Union and its coalition partners. This conflict ultimately led to a government collapse in spring 1993, again bringing health policy reforms to a standstill (see Krajewski-Siuda and Romaniuk 2008).

The next elections, held in 1993, were won by the communist successor party, SLD, who formed a centre-left government coalition with the PSL, with latter's Waldemar Pawlak as Prime Minister. The SLD's victory was seen evidence of the party's success in convincing the Polish electorate that they were not the old communists, but a transformed left party capable of promoting social-democratic values (see Millard 2006). The SLD's position was further strengthened after the 1995 presidential elections, when the party leader Alexander Kwaśniewski won against the incumbent Solidarity leader Lech Wałęsa.

Once in government, the SLD focused on persuading the public of its recently acquired social democratic identity. It rejected the market-oriented proposal prepared by the Social Committee and Solidarity and supported the more statist plan put forward by the inter-ministerial team, seeing it as a better expression of its new social democratic values. The Ministry of Health demonstrated its reform zeal by organising a set of conferences in 1994, with the aim of creating political consensus and developing a technical review of the reform plan. These conferences resulted in a quick transformation of the inter-ministerial proposal into a draft bill, according to which the insurance system would be based on 16 regionally-based insurance funds tasked with negotiating contracts with both public and private healthcare providers. The role of municipal governments in the provider–purchaser relationship would be eliminated, the system would be funded by contributions from both employers and employees at a rate set annually by the Sejm, and the government would provide coverage for the retired and the unemployed.[25]

In December 1994, the bill was presented to the Sejm, with two changes. One was that instead of the shared employer-employee payment of insurance contributions, only employees paid. The other allowed the establishment of additional insurance funds as branch funds of separate industries to allow greater choice and break the regional insurance monopoly. In early 1995, the Council of Ministers approved the bill and returned it to the ministries for consultation; a final draft was submitted to the Sejm in July that year (Bossert and Włodarczyk 2000).

The plans for healthcare reform soon became caught in a political turmoil, however. What initially seemed a stable government coalition

[25] Interview No. 21.

between the SLD and PSL became conflictual. Due to strong inter-coalitional disagreement, dominated by the conflict between PSL Prime Minister Pawlak and SLD leader Alexander Kwaśniewski, in March 1995 Pawlak's government failed after a vote of no confidence. A new government was formed under a renewed coalition agreement between the two parties with Józef Oleksy from SLD as Prime Minister.

In the meantime, the opposition criticised the government's proposal as overly statist and put forward an alternative, market-oriented reform plan. The opposition's plan was based on the earlier proposals of the Social Committee and Solidarity and was submitted for discussion in the Sejm by President Lech Wałęsa in August 1995. Instead of a regionally organised insurance system, this plan opted for a competitive insurance market based on independent funds. Given the stark differences between the two proposals and the threat that Wałęsa would use his presidential powers to veto the law based on the government reform plan, an Extraordinary Committee of the Sejm was appointed to find a compromise.

Compromise was difficult, hampered by another re-shuffling of the government due to Oleksy's resignation and the appointment of Włodzimierz Cimoszewicz (SLD) as Prime Minister. In December 1995, the SLD's position was strengthened by the defeat of Wałęsa and the election of Kwaśniewski as President. The Sejm's Extraordinary Committee presented a draft of a new healthcare insurance bill, which basically retained the original ideas from the inter-ministerial proposal, leaving very limited scope for competition. The bill introduced a regional health insurance system based on employee contributions, which amounted to 10 per cent of wages, and 16 regional insurance funds plus one branch fund for the uniformed forces. It also stipulated that these funds would be given significant financial and political independence, and envisaged creation of an 'equalisation fund' to even out the risk differences amongst clients of different funds. Suggesting the SLD's ideological flexibility and the party's willingness to demonstrate its pro-reformist identity (see Grzymała-Busse 2002), the bill proposed consideration of additional private insurance funds a year after the new insurance was set in place. Because the government had a majority, the bill was passed in the Sejm, supported in the Senate, and then returned to the Sejm where it was finally approved and signed by the President as the 1997 Law on Healthcare Insurance.[26]

[26] Usta*wa o powszechnym ubezpieczeniu zdrowotnym*, Law No. 28/153.

Shift Towards Managed Competition

Introduction of the 1997 insurance law was not the closing chapter of healthcare financing reform. The September 1997 elections resulted in the comeback of the Solidarity block with the victory of Solidarity Electoral Action (AWS) and was a major setback for the incumbent parties, the PSL and SLD. The new government formed by a centrist liberal coalition between the AWS and another liberal party, the Freedom Union (UW), under AWS leader Jerzy Buzek, was a stable majority government and the first Polish post-communist government to serve its full term.

Buzek's government had an extraordinary chance to change the healthcare financing reform, as implementation of the 1997 Law on Healthcare Insurance was scheduled for January 1999. It had been delayed because of the need to coordinate health reform with the parallel reform of public administration that divided Poland into three administrative levels: voivodeships (*województwa*), counties (*powiats*), and municipalities (*gminas*). The idea was that the delay in the implementation of the new insurance system should leave enough time to develop the administrative infrastructure needed to establish the regional insurance funds.

The Ministry of Health under Buzek published a reform document suggesting changes to the 1997 Law on Health Insurance that involved more strongly market-oriented elements, based on Solidarity's 1993 reform proposal. This new proposal was designed by actors who were very fond of market solutions and strongly driven by their beliefs and 'ideological views'.[27] Appointing Teresa Kamińska, the co-author of the original Solidarity proposal, as the Minister in charge of Social Policy Coordination was meant to strengthen the AWS's power position in the area of welfare reforms (Bossert and Włodarczyk 2000).[28] However, the strong pro-market orientation was partly counterbalanced by the UW's appointment of former Finance Minister Leszek Balcerowicz as Deputy Prime Minister. In a rather strange contrast to his sturdy neo-liberal, pro-market views of economic reform, Balcerowicz (1995) advocated a moderate approach to healthcare (McMenamin and Timonen 2002; see also Sitek 2008). He wanted to balance the healthcare budget and reduce the sector's financial deficit and was therefore against the idea of private health insurance and unregulated doctor's fees. He believed the introduction of the strongly

[27] Interview No. 21.

[28] Interview No. 21.

competitive fee-for-service format suggested in the Solidarity proposal would only cause additional financial problems in an already vulnerable sector (Bossert and Włodarczyk 1999).

In April 1998, the Ministry presented a bill to amend the 1997 law. It was a clear result of Balcerowicz's influence and a compromise between the AWS and the UW. The bill called for the reduction of healthcare insurance contributions to 7.5 per cent of wages. This was an important victory for the UW and Balcerowitz, as during the election campaign, the AWS promised to increase contributions, and the proposed reductions were the result of pressure from the Deputy Prime Minister. In terms of competition, the bill stipulated that whilst regional insurance funds would be maintained, there would be room for competition between branch funds (Bossert and Włodarczyk 1999), and additional insurance funds could enter the health insurance market in 2002 (*Gazeta Wyborcza* 2000).

In addition, instead of a general ballot, the board of regional insurance funds would be elected by newly established *voivodeship* parliaments, and contributions would be collected not by local governments, but by the state agency responsible for social insurance, the Social Insurance Fund, and then transferred from this central fund to the insurance funds. The bill also reduced doctors' decision-making power by eliminating direct negotiations between the insurance funds and the professional associations and replacing these with negotiations between the funds and the local governments. The political power over the insurance system was further strengthened by an additional provision putting the regional assemblies in charge of appointing the funds' management members.

These provisions were passed into law as the 1998 Amendment to the Law on Health Insurance.[29] The AWS's concessions to Balcerowicz's demands made the amendment's passing in the Sejm relatively easy. The only possible threat was the veto of President Kwaśniewski, who was from SLD and, as such, belonged to the old unreformed communists. Yet, Kwaśniewski's veto power was weakened; the 1997 changes to the Polish Constitution had reduced presidential powers, and the President's veto could be overturned by a 60 per cent vote in the Sejm (Millard 2000). Even though the AWS-UW coalition did not have the 276 deputies needed to overthrow the President's veto, the coalition had broken Kwaśniewski's vetoes in the past by finding allies in the opposition (*Dziennik Polski*

[29] *Ustawa z dnia 18 lipca 1998 r. o zmianie ustawy o powszechnym ubezpieczeniu zdrowotnym oraz o zmianie niektórych ustaw*, Law No. 117/756.

2005). As chances of his veto being rejected were high, and Kwaśniewski was also known as someone who 'rarely fought battles he could not win' (McMenamin 2008), he signed the amendment after its passage in Parliament.

The Polish doctors, unsurprisingly, strongly opposed the amendments. They openly criticised the new system, saying the management of the insurance funds by regional assemblies was a sign of political influence and control over financial decisions in the healthcare sector. They further claimed the new health insurance system was poorly designed and criticised aspects of the reform architecture, such as the low levels of insurance contributions, the lack of guaranteed contracting for service providers, and the elimination of direct negotiations between the funds and the professional associations.[30] To voice their opposition, the Polish Doctors Trade Union, together with other associations of doctors and medical workers, established the Committee for the Defence of Health Reform (*Komitet Obrony Reformy Zdrowia*) with the aim of protesting the implementation of the health insurance system (OZZL 2022). However, the doctors' opposition was futile, suggesting the impact of professional interests on major health reforms followed alternative channels and remained insignificant, in contradiction to the claims of some scholars (see Roberts 2009).

Shift Towards Centralised Health Insurance

Despite the doctors' protests, the new insurance system was implemented. It quickly faced multiple problems, however. For example, healthcare reform was one reform in a set of large-scale public sector reforms. These other reforms involved three major sectors—public administration, pensions, and education—and the four large reforms were to be implemented simultaneously, starting on 1 January 1999. Of the four, the healthcare reform was considered the riskiest to implement, as the amendment to the 1997 law was passed just a few months before the scheduled implementation and still required significant clarification of its regulations.[31]

Other implementation problems were administrative. Because of the regionally structured nature of the insurance system, implementation of the Law on Healthcare Insurance and its amendments depended on the

[30] *Gazeta Lekarska* 1998 No. 4.
[31] Interview No. 22.

simultaneous implementation of the public administration reform. This latter reform created a new territorial division of the country with the creation of 16 regions and initiated the administrative and electoral process necessary for the implementation of the new, regionally-based health insurance system. Even though the two reforms were coordinated on paper, their legislation was not consistent and required additional regulations to be put in place (Bossert and Włodarczyk 1999).

Further inconsistencies occurred, as the health insurance legislation contradicted one of the major laws on public administration, the 1995 Law on Large Cities.[32] This law gave some municipalities a strong role in the ownership and management of healthcare provision at the local level, allowing them to decide whether healthcare services would be delivered by public or private providers. The 1997 Law on Health Insurance curtailed this role by delegating it to the newly established health insurance funds, thus leaving municipalities to play a role only in the ownership of public facilities and participation in the government of the insurance funds. Besides being an administrative issue, these coordination problems generated obstacles for patients, who, especially during the initial stages of the reform, had difficulty understanding where (in which hospitals and health centres) they could get care and who would cover the costs of the services (Bossert and Włodarczyk 1999: 15–17).

Another set of problems emerged due to the lack of managerial capacity in the context of quasi-markets in the insurance sector, generating examples of market failures. The 1997 law called for insurance contributions to be collected by the government, transferred to the Social Insurance Fund, and transferred from there to the 16 regions plus one branch insurance funds. As might be expected, this new and complicated system of financing quickly caused confusion. The financing system was complex, and a variety of different, regionally specific and often competitive reimbursement schemes were now in play. As the insurance funds were autonomous, they were able to decide which specific schemes they would like to use in their region, that is, their branch. However, this complicated the job of the Social Insurance Fund; it proved incapable of tracking the different schemes and distributing the insurance contributions accordingly. This led to delays in money transfers and risked insurance funds becoming insolvent; the government had to break the law by providing loans to help the

[32] *Ustawa z dnia 24 listopada 1995 r. o zmianie zakresu działania niektórych miast oraz o miejskich strefach usług publicznych.*

system going. At the same time, as most funds introduced competitive reimbursement schemes or opted for experimental combinations of different schemes, they started to overspend, generating additional financial losses in the system (see McMenamin and Timonen 2002). To prevent the system from running into serious financial difficulties, the government passed an additional amendment to the 1997 law, raising the contribution level from 7.5 per cent to 7.75 per cent and scheduling a 0.25 per cent annual increase in the contribution rate, thus triggering a gradual increase in the contribution level.[33]

Final problems were political, as the 1998 amendment to the Law on Health Insurance had assigned significant powers to the local level. The local governments now owned most of the public healthcare facilities and were able to select managerial staff for the regional healthcare insurance funds. As a result of this political influence, the funds became subject to the interests of political parties. The parties, which were weakly institutionalised and had little to offer to their members in terms of material incentives and support, started to see the local governments as a vital source of 'jobs for the boys' (see Filinson et al. 2003). Because of these political appointees, the funds quickly became more interested in satisfying their constituents than implementing the intended reform goals.

During the troubled implementation of the new insurance system, one of the key disputes was the introduction of private insurance companies, scheduled for 2002. This plan was discussed by the government's coalition partners, and because of the implementation problems, they considered postponing the entry of private insurance companies to 2005. The SLD, at this time an opposition party, feared the commercial health insurance funds would use advertising and additional insurance packages to attract the young, the healthy, and the rich, leaving the poor, sick, and the elderly in the public insurance system. This risked creating a division between the rich and the poor and would have a significant effect on the accessibility of healthcare services. However, government experts such as Teresa Kamińska, now the advisor to the Prime Minister, argued cream-skimming could be prevented by not allowing private funds to select their clients and by financially equalising the funds. More generally, Kamińska said the entry of private insurance companies and competition would be crucial for

[33] *Ustawa z dnia 30 listopada 2000 r. o zmianie ustawy o powszechnym ubezpieczeniu zdrowotnym*, Law No. 122/1311.

health system reform, as it would provide a necessary stimulus to finally 'put the health system in order' (*Gazeta Wyborcza* 2000).

Unsurprisingly, given the multiple implementation problems, the health insurance system was unpopular amongst doctors and the wider public. The doctors continued to voice their opposition to the new system through protests, strikes, and a refusal to fill out the required forms for the insurance funds.[34] Anaesthesiologists, organised around the Anaesthesiologist Trade Union, went on a hunger strike, refusing to sign contracts with the insurance funds and demanding to continue signing direct contracts with the *voivodeship* for the provision of their services. To demonstrate their opposition to the new system, the Committee for the Defence of Health Reform organised a general two-hour strike of healthcare services in January 1999, but this had little effect (OZZL 2022). Public opinion polls suggested the wider public was similarly dissatisfied. A nation-wide opinion survey carried out one year after the implementation of the insurance system showed many Poles were dissatisfied with the healthcare sector. Seventy-nine per cent of respondents thought the system was malfunctioning, and 6 per cent considered the state of the healthcare sector worse than before the reform (CBOS 2000; see also Rincker and Battle 2011).

The deeply unpopular health reform became a key issue in the 2001 election campaign. Building on the strong negative perception of the reform, as part of its electoral platform, the SLD, running in coalition with the smaller leftist Labour Union (*Unia Pracy—UP*), proposed abolition of the 16 regional insurance funds, arguing they should be replaced by a smaller number of bigger funds (Krajewski-Siuda and Romaniuk 2008).[35] This proposal became one of the points of the coalition's electoral campaign and contributed to its winning more than 40 per cent of all votes in Sejm, whilst the SLD won a convincing majority in the Senate, thus marking a big comeback of the communist successor parties. This was coupled with the political extinction of the AWS, that is, the Solidarity block, which failed to win any votes (Szczerbiak 2002; Millard 2003, 2009).

Following the elections, the SLD-UP coalition formed a majority government with a smaller party (PSL) under Leszek Miller as Prime Minister. Miller appointed Marius Łapinski, an SLD member and a controversial figure, as Minister of Health. As soon as he took the ministerial position,

[34] *Gazeta Lekarska* 1998 No. 9.

[35] Interview No. 25.

Łapinski put forward a radical proposal to abolish the regional insurance system and replace it with a single health insurance fund governed directly by the state. The ministerial proposal represented a U-turn towards centralisation, as this fund, to be called the National Health Fund (*Narodowy Fundus Zdrowia—NFZ*), would feature regional branches with a very limited range of organisational functions.[36] Responsibility for the preparation of health plans, used as a basis for the contracting of health services, would be held by the Minister of Health, thus significantly limiting the range of choice amongst local decision makers.[37] Finally, Łapinski's reform proposal called for direct political supervision of the NFZ by the Fund Council, composed of nine members appointed by the Prime Minister for a five-year period (Kuszewski et al. 2005: 11).

To justify re-centralisation, Minister Łapinski claimed the health reform implemented by the liberal AWS-UW government resulted in the Ministry of Health's loss of control and showed its incapacity to create state healthcare policy. Clearly favouring the paradigm of a state-run health system, Łapinski argued a centralised financing of healthcare services was better able to ensure efficiency and equality of health provision than a competitive system of multiple health insurance funds. The reform was needed, he said, and the collapsing insurance system left no room for compromise. Re-centralisation was necessary to save the system and avoid bankruptcy (Łapinski 2003).

Łapinski's proposal was strongly criticised by healthcare experts and the post-Solidarity parties, now in opposition. Amongst the public, the idea of the healthcare re-centralisation also attracted relatively little support, with more than 30 per cent of the respondents in a public opinion survey agreeing that centralising the health system was not the solution to its problems (CBOS 2001). A related survey showed significant public disquiet, with almost half of all respondents (46 per cent) claiming they were dissatisfied with the healthcare system as a whole (CBOS 2002). The only support for re-centralisation came from a specific sub-group of doctors who were directors of hospital wards. They supported Łapinski's reform, hoping it would allow them to regain part of the control they had lost in the context

[36] Interview No. 24.
[37] Interview No. 20.

of a competitive insurance system.[38] Despite the opposition, Miller's government decided to approve the Minister's reform proposal, seeing it as a way to reduce public dissatisfaction.[39] The government had a majority in the Sejm, the SLD dominated the Senate, and party member Kwaśniewski was still in the presidential role—this combination strongly suggested any potential vetoes would be ineffective. Accordingly, the government introduced re-centralisation in the 2003 Law on Health Insurance with the National Health Fund.[40]

The problems did not disappear, however, and in the first few months of its existence, the National Health Fund generated further reasons for discontent. One of the many issues in the functioning of the Fund was that the centralised organisation of the insurance system did not solve the problem of inefficiency in the distribution of healthcare resources, and this continued to plague the sector. Another issue was political influence on the governance of the Fund; this led to major instabilities marked by frequent changes of the Fund's personnel and presidents (Krajewski-Siuda and Romaniuk 2008). In the context of increasing dissatisfaction with the health system and with the government as a whole, accompanied by a decrease in support for the SLD, Miller's government dismissed Health Minister Łapinski and replaced him with Marek Balicki in January 2003. Far from solving the problem, however, this initiated a series of ministerial replacements, signalling a government crisis and highlighting its weak leadership in the health sector.[41]

The strongest opposition to the new setup of the Polish health system came from primary care physicians. Arguing that the contract conditions of the National Health Fund were extremely unfavourable for primary health providers, they organised a large anti-government protest causing an almost total paralysis of the healthcare system (Pilonis 2004). Hoping to tame the opposition of medical professionals, the Ministry of Health initiated a Round Table on Health Care in June 2003. By then, however,

[38] In the context of the competitive insurance system instituted in 1999, regional insurance funds were able to reject contracts with hospitals; this restricted hospitals' power, including the power of the directors of hospital wards (Interview No. 24).

[39] Interview No. 24.

[40] *Ustawa o powszechnym ubezpieczeniu w Narodowym Funduszu Zdrowia*, Law. No. 45/391.

[41] Balicki was replaced by Leszek Sikorski in April 2003, and in May 2004, Sikorski was replaced by Wojciech Rudnicki. After just 17 days, Rudnicki was replaced by Marian Czakański.

it was already too late to secure support for the reforms, and they were widely opposed in professional circles (Krajewski-Siuda and Romaniuk 2008). Within the political opposition, the PO became the most vocal party criticising the 2003 law; amongst other things, the PO argued the law was implemented too quickly, the provisions lacked clarity, and the centralisation of the insurance system violated the rights of the insured (*Gazeta Wyborcza* 2003).

The overall discontent with the new setup of the health system culminated in January 2004, when the legality of the 2003 law came under the scrutiny of the Polish Constitutional Court. A group of MPs from the PO challenged the law and asked the Court to check its constitutionality. After consideration, the Court determined the 2003 law was inconsistent with an article of the Constitution granting health protection, established only fictitious freedom of providers' choice for patients, and generated confusion about patients' entitlements. The Court also said the law did not grant any real control powers to the insured and did not even ensure proper supervision of the National Health Fund by the Minister of Health. It asked the government to repeal the problematic parts of the law and amend it in accordance with the constitutional provisions by the end of 2004 (Polish Constitutional Court 2004; see also *Gazeta Wyborcza* 2003, 2004a).

Following the Court's request, the government decided to revoke the 2003 law and started working on a new piece of legislation. The debate on the new law was lively, with all parties suggesting different reform ideas. The liberal PO proposed the introduction of private health insurance, but was criticised by another opposition party, the conservative PiS, who favoured a publicly funded system (*Gazeta Wyborca* 2004b). The result of the debate was the 2004 Law on Health Care Services Financed from Public Sources.[42] This law introduced a few key changes in response to the Court's decision, but left the National Health Insurance fund in place, thus keeping the centralised structure of the insurance system untouched. In response to the demand to clarify patients' entitlements and provide stronger control over the system, the law introduced a 'negative' list of services, that is, services not financed by the Fund, and established more transparent regulations in the management of waiting lists for scheduled interventions and hospitalisations. It also made important changes in the governance of the Fund, abolishing its Board and thus reducing its

[42] *Ustawa o świadczeniach opieki zdrowotnej finansowanych ze środków publicznych*, Law No. 210/2135.

susceptibility to political influence. However, the new law did not increase the independence of the Fund's regional branches, leaving the centralised and essentially monopsonic model of health insurance in place (Kuszewski et al. 2005: 13).

Attempts to Return to Managed Competition

The constitutional debate over the 2003 law on National Health Fund just added to the general feeling that Miller's government was incompetent in the area of healthcare policy, and its reform attempts were as ineffective as those of its discredited predecessor (Szczerbiak 2007). In this context, it was unsurprising that the results of the September 2005 elections signalled the political demise of the left and generated a new round of reform. Despite its optimistic electoral slogan 'We have changed, now we can change Poland' (Millard 2006), SLD failed dramatically, losing almost 30 per cent of its parliamentary power. The conservative PiS and the liberal PO gained the highest shares of votes.

The PiS and PO had divergent views on health reform, and this had been evident during the debate over the constitutionality of the 2003 law on Nationa Health Fund. Their electoral platforms in the 2005 elections further underlined their differences. PiS emphasised the constitutional right of every citizen to health protection, equity and equality of healthcare access, and the principle of social solidarity (PiS 2005). The party's reform vision included the abolition of the insurance system, a return to financing health from the state budget, and a clear definition of the healthcare services guaranteed by the state. The PO proposed a significantly more market-oriented plan (Klepka 2008). This plan included a system based on multiple, competitive insurance funds and the establishment of a Health System Supervisory Authority who would oversee the financial stability of the funds and their compliance with the standards set by the Minister of Health. It also promised the creation of an Agency for Standardisation and Tariffs, a central government body subordinate to the Ministry, in charge of modifying the basket of health benefits financed by public funds. Finally, it offered to introduce private health insurance, stressing the need for mechanisms that would not jeopardise the financial sustainability of the public health funds.

After the 2005 elections, the PiS formed a government with other two parties, the populist agrarian Self-defence of the Republic of Poland (SRP) and the conservative League of Polish Families (LPR) under Kazimierz

Marcinkiewicz. The Ministry of Health led by Zbigniew Religa put forward a reform proposal which essentially broke the party's electoral promises. Arguing for the abolition of the NFZ, instead of making a switch to budget financing, it proposed to introduce multiple competitive insurance funds. The idea of a competitive insurance system was not supported by the other two parties in the governing coalition, the SRP and LRP. However, the PO, the largest opposition party, declared it was ready to support the government plan, thus creating a potential reform coalition of the two parties. The PiS, however, decided to follow the coalition agreement and abandoned the plan.

PiS's idea to replace the NFZ with a system financed by the state budget re-emerged in 2016, when the party returned to power in a coalition with other conservative-right parties under Beata Szydło as Prime Minister. The Health Ministry, led by Konstanty Radziwiłł, presented a reform document titled, 'Strategy for changes in the health care system', which emphasised free healthcare for all, a budget financing system, and possibly a mixed system with a combination of a public, tax-financed system and private insurance (*Gazeta Prawna* 2015). However, this plan was very controversial, was criticised as underdeveloped, and was abandoned by the government in 2017, with the party suggesting the abolition of the NFZ was a matter for the 'next term in office' (*Gazeta Prawna* 2017).

Attempts to Introduce Private Health Insurance

The 2005 government plans for a return to managed competition may have suggested possible agreement between the two largest, right-wing political entities, the PO and the PiS, but the following period was marked by increasing inter-party conflict. After the fall of the PiS government in 2007, the 2007 elections resulted in the PO's victory and a new right-wing government, but this time based on a coalition between the PO and the agrarian Christian-democratic Polish People Party (PSL), under Donald Tusk as the Prime Minister. In early 2008, the Tusk government, with the Ministry of Health led by Ewa Kopacz, initiated the 'White Summit' consultations to discuss health system reform priorities with stakeholders, including representatives of trade unions, local authorities, and patient groups. The outcome was a list of reforms, officially published as the Ministry of Health's legislative priorities for future reform, even though they were not approved by the largest trade unions. This list contained no less than 16 laws and 41 decrees. The dramatic, large-scale change of the health system would include the introduction of supplementary private healthcare insurance and hospital privatisation, but also strengthen patient rights (*Gazeta Prawna* 2010a).

One of the key elements of the reform plan was the introduction of private insurance. Private health insurance was already available for those not insured by the NFZ, such as migrants, or for those wanting access to private providers (Popic 2021b). In this context, the PO's plan was to provide a legal framework to make the use of private insurance easier and put it on an equal standing with public insurance, leading to a tighter public-private mix. These plans were not new. One result of the PO's constitutional challenge of the 2003 law had been the definition of the 'negative' services, or services not covered by public health insurance. Minister Kopacz argued the 'negative list' was important: it was an indirect definition of services belonging to the basic benefit package, and as such, it would strengthen patients' rights, providing them with knowledge on the type of services to which they were entitled (*Rynek Zdrowia* 2008a). Defining this negative list was also considered crucial to prepare the ground for the introduction of private insurance, as it clearly delineated competences for the public health system and for potential private providers (Holly and Szczepaniak 2011).

Demonstrating it was eager to push for private markets in health insurance, Kopacz's Ministry submitted a bill to the Sejm even before the 'White Summit' consultation. The bill proposed introducing two types of insurance. One was complementary, to cover services which were not or only partially covered by the public insurance system, that is, services requiring co-payments and services on the 'negative list'. The other was supplementary insurance to allow higher quality of service or faster access to services within the public system. The complementary insurance coverage would enable patients, for example, to choose a date on which they wished to be operated or have a hospital room of a higher standard. It would also allow for choice of doctors and additional nursing care, and would cover diagnostic tests, dental treatments, and visits to specialists. The bill proposed the introduction of tax breaks for private insurance, giving tax relief by deducting the contribution for private insurance from personal income. In addition, employers would be able to finance contributions to private insurance from companies' funds for welfare benefits. Overall, the idea was that tax breaks and possibilities for employers to use private health insurance as a fringe benefit for their employees would contribute to the growth of private insurance (Kopacz 2008; see also *Gazeta Prawna* 2008a).

During the parliamentary discussion, the bill on private insurance was criticised as underdeveloped and not in line with the existing legislation, as the latter did not have a precise definition of services covered by public insurance. Minister Kopacz herself admitted that the bill needed elaboration. She said that to proceed, they needed, in addition to the 'negative list', a more precise definition of the basic benefit package (Kopacz 2008). As a result, the proposal was withdrawn in April 2008.

Following this failure, the Ministry of Health started working hard on the definition of basic benefit package. The PiS, the largest opposition party, argued against this policy measure, claiming the definition of benefits partly or fully covered by public insurance would permit private healthcare financing to enter through the 'back door'. The PiS leader, President Lech Kaczyński, expressed strong doubts about the idea of a basic benefit package, suggesting the Ministry's initiatives risked legislative failure due to a possible presidential veto. Kopacz nevertheless proposed a bill on amendments to the Law on Health Services Financed from the Public Funds. It passed in Parliament and was signed by the President. Kaczyński's decision not to veto the law on the benefit package was seen as surprising, but could be explained by the fact that he was simply being strategic, as he saw another imminent policy issue, hospital privatisation (see next section), gave him the possibility for a much wider disagreement with Kopacz's reform plan (*Rynek Zdrowia* 2009).

The newly defined basic benefit package enabled Kopacz's Ministry to make another attempt to introduce private insurance in 2011. The new bill on private insurance, in contrast to the 2008 proposal, proposed three insurance types—complementary, supplementary, and substitute insurance—where substitute insurance would be an alternative for those not obliged to pay a contribution to the NFZ. The aim of the reform, as stated by the Ministry of Health, was faster access to benefits financed by the NFZ and higher standards of providing benefits and services not covered by public insurance. This, in turn, aimed at increasing competition between public and private insurance to improve patients' choice. Like the previous bill on private insurance, this one included tax breaks for private health insurance and the possibility of financing contributions for this insurance from company funds (Jurkiewicz-Świętek 2012).

As soon as the bill was submitted for consultation, it encountered strong criticism. One complaint was that the change in the insurance structure would hit the most vulnerable. Minister Kopacz argued this would not happen, as a protection mechanism would be in place (Kopacz 2010). Supporting the Minister, Deputy Minister of Health Jakub Szulc argued that in practice the introduction of private insurance would not be a significant change; Poles, he said, were already paying privately to access healthcare services outside the public system. Introducing private insurance would simply eliminate these 'double payments' and help regulate the flow of private sources spent on healthcare, estimated at between 22 and 30 billion per year (*Gazeta Prawna* 2010b). In another attack on the proposed bill, Minister of Finance Jacek Rostowski challenged the idea of introducing tax breaks for private insurance. Kopacz claimed that without these breaks, private health insurance would remain undeveloped, but Rostowski warned the provision risked being contrary to the Law on Public Finance, limiting the government's ability to adopt bills with a possible negative impact on the public budget (*Rynek Zdrowia* 2010). After facing a barrage of criticism over private insurance and simultaneously waging a heated political debate on the proposed hospital reform (see next section), the Ministry ultimately abandoned the bill on the introduction of private insurance.

Attempt to Privatise Hospitals

As in other countries of the former Eastern Bloc, hospital transformation in Poland was not a significant policy issue during the early transitional period, as major attention was given to the creation of an insurance-based system of healthcare financing. However, when the country's insurance system was set in place, privatisation of public hospitals became a salient issue within the broader reform paradigm of marketisation. The issue of hospital privatisation deeply divided the two right-wing parties, the liberal PO and the conservative PiS. PiS party leader Lech Kaczyński was President and, as such, had veto powers. This meant the PiS could block the government's plans to turn Poland's public hospitals into commercial companies.

The plans for the privatisation of public hospitals took concrete shape in the first Tusk government under Kopacz's Ministry.[43] The list of the government's reform priorities, announced after the 'White Summit'

[43] The first concrete proposal to privatise hospitals appeared in 2001, under the AWS-UW government but was quickly withdrawn because of the breakdown of the governing coalition and the upcoming elections (Kaczmarek et al. 2013).

consultations, contained a provision whereby hospitals would be given more autonomy and transformed into limited liability or joint-stock companies, governed by commercial law. Hospital transformation became the most controversial topic in the broader reform debate, largely because of the poor financial situation of the hospital sector, organised at that time through Autonomous Public Healthcare Units (*Samodzielny publiczny zakład opieki zdrowotnej*—SPZOZ) and characterised by a large and growing debt. Arguing the hospital system needed a new legal framework and a more efficient management model, the government proposed the obligatory transformation of all SPZOZs into limited liability joint-stock companies. The main aim was not to privatise hospitals but to improve their financial management and end the process of uncontrolled indebtedness (*Gazeta Wyborcza* 2008).

The bill for the privatisation of hospitals became a part of a broader reform package of the Kopacz Ministry, containing four laws: Bill on Patients' Rights, Bill on Provisions Introducing Laws in the Field of Health Protection, Bill on Employees of Healthcare Institutions, and Bill on Healthcare Facilities, the last of which envisaged hospital transformation into joint-stock companies. Kopacz's reform package was attacked by the PiS, with PiS's former Minister of Health, Zbigniew Religa one of its most vocal opponents. Religa argued the government's plan was not a reform but an anti-reform, because it left out the patient. Speaking against the Law on Healthcare Facilities, Religa stated:

> As a doctor for many years, I see a huge threat to the Polish health service in the implementation of this reform. A private hospital looks beautiful, but there are no loss-making wards, for example the emergency ones. Therefore, commercialisation is the worst thing for the patient. Everywhere, in the entire old European Union. European medical aid is based on public medicine, not on commercialised medicine. (Religa, cited in Sowińska 2010)

Another key figure attacking the reform plans was the PiS leader, President Lech Kaczyński. In consultation with Religia and another of PiS's former Ministers of Health, Marek Balicki, Kaczyński came up with the idea of holding a national referendum on the privatisation of hospitals after the legislation was passed. The referendum was meant to ask citizens whether they agreed 'to the commercialisation of healthcare facilities, which will enable the privatisation of hospitals'. However, this referendum proposal was rejected by the Senate, at that time dominated by the PO.

The debate over hospital reform reached another peak in July 2008 when the PiS put forward a vote of no confidence in Kopacz as Minister of Health. This failed but generated further tensions between the two parties (*Rynek Zdrowia* 2008b). The conflict between the PO and PiS became even more tense in November 2008 when, thanks to the government's parliamentary majority, the Sejm approved Kopacz's reform package. As a last resort, Kaczyński decided to use his presidential powers. Vetoing all but one law from the reform package (Law on Patients' Rights) on 27 November, the President said he was vetoing the plan for obligatory commercialisation of public hospitals because it compromised citizens' health. More specifically, in his opinion, the most problematic element of the proposed reform was that it contradicted the principle of solidarity in access to health services (Kaczyński 2008). The vetoed healthcare laws now faced a re-vote in the Sejm. Kopacz said she would do everything possible to block support of the veto, arguing the President had exaggerated the government plans: 'he created a dragon of the alleged privatisation of hospitals, such as if it breathes fire and devours patients' (*Gazeta Prawna* 2008b). Kaczyński's veto was successful, however, as the opponents of the veto did not get the majority required to reject it in the Sejm.

Following the presidential veto, the government decided to introduce hospitals' transformation through the 'back door' by leaving changes up to local governments. In February 2009, the Tusk government presented a new programme, 'Save Polish Hospitals', which aimed to offer assistance to local authorities who were converting hospitals into commercial companies. The implementation was supposed to be coordinated by the Ministry of Health and the NFZ, and supported by an appointed expert group. The plan had limited success, however, as the local governments were not very eager for hospital transformation. By 2010, only a small portion of public hospitals had become joint-stock companies (Żukowski 2013).

Poland's political landscape was shaken in 2010 by the sudden death of President Lech Kaczyński in the Smolensk air crash. The subsequent presidential elections resulted in the victory of the PO's vice-chairman, Bronisław Komorowski; he defeated Jarosłav Kaczyński, twin brother of the deceased President and chairman of the PiS. In this new political and institutional configuration, the Tusk government engaged in yet another attempt to indirectly privatise Polish hospitals, passing the Law on

Healthcare Activities in 2011.[44] With a clear intention to indirectly transform public hospitals, this law stipulated that local governments would take on responsibility to cover debts of public healthcare facilities; if they were not able to do so, they would be obliged to transform the indebted facilities into either companies governed by the commercial code, that is, limited liability or joint-stock companies, or budgetary units. Whilst one of the law's main objectives was to abolish the legal form of the SPZOZs, the new type of legal transformation did not necessarily imply liquidation and the takeover of all the facilities' liabilities by the local government (Mikuła and Kaczmarek 2019). To motivate the local governments to take part in this transformation, the government offered financial support for hospitals deciding to convert before the end of 2013 (Sagan and Sobczak 2014).

In an attempt to oppose the plan, PiS again tried to remove Minister Kopacz from the office, again unsuccessfully (*Rynek Zdrowia* 2011). Yet, independently of PiS opposition, the full-scale hospital transformation was slow and protracted. By mid-2013, only 33 facilities had been transformed into limited liability or joint-stock companies, including 22 hospitals and 11 ambulatory healthcare units, with only about 30 more planned for that year.

Local governments who owned hospitals were reluctant to transform them into commercial companies for several reasons. They preferred to commercialise facilities that were in good financial condition and more likely to survive the conversion, whilst providing financial support to those in poor condition to avoid their mandatory transformation. Moreover, although the local governments were still legally obliged to provide healthcare to the population, transformation implied they would lose control of the commercialised hospitals. Lastly, there were doubts about the benefits of commercialisation, especially for those hospitals in good financial condition (Sagan and Sobczak 2014). As a result, the process of indirect hospital transformation was not very successful; commercialisation affected only 18 per cent of all the hospitals in the country (Mikuła and Kaczmarek 2019).

[44] *Ustawa o działalności leczniczej*, Law No. 112/654.

Conclusion

This chapter has accounted for the Polish health policy developments in post-communism, marked by *reversals* and failures, a pattern which contrasts with the Slovenian *survival* and the Czech *instability* of market-oriented reforms. It has analysed the key policy episodes driving the development of this peculiar policy path and accounted for the factors shaping it. The lack of policy experience with markets in healthcare under socialism and the turbulent politics of the early transition, notably the conflict between the communist successor party and the anti-communist post-Solidarity parties, were key factors in the delayed introduction of a de-centralised and competitive insurance system and the subsequent large-scale policy reversal. The gradual disappearance of the successor parties from the political scene was coupled with the emergence of a new conflict centred on the issue of hospital privatisation between the two right-wing parties, one with a conservative and another with a liberal orientation. The recurring pattern of strong party divisions over the core health reforms and an institutional arrangement of thick veto configurations made it difficult to adapt market ideas and protracted the process of policy learning.

References

Balcerowicz, Leszek. 1995. *Socialism, capitalism, transformation.* Budapest: Central European University Press.

Barr, Nicholas A. 1994. *Labor markets and social policy in Central and Eastern Europe: The transition and beyond.* Washington, DC: World Bank Publications.

Bossert, Thomas, and W. Cezary Włodarczyk. 2000. *Unpredictable politics: Policy process of health reform in Poland.* International Health System Program, Harvard School of Public Health. Accessed 18 December 2021. http://www.hsph.harvard.edu/ihsg/publications/pdf/No-74.PDF.

CBOS. 2000. *Opinie o opiece zdrowotnej* [Opinions about healthcare]. Centrum Badania Opinii Społezney. Accessed 4 January 2022. https://cbos.pl/SPISKOM.POL/2000/K_019_00.PDF.

———. 2001. *Critical opinion on the effects of the health care reform.* Centrum Badania Opinii Społezney. Accessed 4 January 2022. http://www.cbos.pl/PL/publikacje/public_opinion/2000/12_2000.pdf.

———. 2002. *Opinions on healthcare in Poland.* Centrum Badania Opinii Społezney. Accessed 4 January 2022. https://www.cbos.pl/PL/publikacje/public_opinion/2002/10_2002.pdf.

Cerami, Alfio. 2006. *Social policy in Central and Eastern Europe: The emergence of a new European welfare regime*. Münster: LIT Verlag.

Constitution of the Republic of Poland. 1997. Accessed 23 December 2021. https://www.constituteproject.org/constitution/Poland_1997.pdf.

Dziennik Polski. 2005. *Prezydenckie weta* [Presidential vetoes]. Accessed 27 December 2021. https://dziennikpolski24.pl/prezydenckie-weta/ar/1598902.

Ekiert, Grzegorz, and Jan Kubik. 2001. *Rebellious civil society: Popular protest and democratic consolidation in Poland, 1989–1993*. Ann Arbor: University of Michigan Press.

Elster, Jon. 1996. *The roundtable talks and the breakdown of communism*. Chicago: University of Chicago Press.

Filinson, Rachel, Piotr Chmielewski, and Darek Niklas. 2003. Back to the future: Polish health care reform. *Communist and Post-Communist Studies* 36 (4): 385–403.

Gazeta Prawna. 2008a. *Resort zdrowia ma nowy projekt ustawy o dodatkowych ubezpieczeniach zdrowotnych* [The Ministry of Health has a new bill on additional health insurance], 11 September. Accessed 10 January 2022. https://praca.gazetaprawna.pl/artykuly/35308,resort-zdrowia-ma-nowy-projekt-ustawy-o-dodatkowych-ubezpieczeniach-zdrowotnych.html.

———. 2008b. *Sejm za wetem prezydenta do ustaw zdrowotnych* [Sejm for the president's veto on health bills]. Accessed 20 January 2022. https://praca.gazetaprawna.pl/artykuly/101565,sejm-za-wetem-prezydenta-do-ustaw-zdrowotnych.html.

———. 2010a. *Minister Kopacz ma nowy pomysł na reformę służby zdrowia* [Minister Kopacz has a new idea for the health care reform], 28 February. Accessed 10 January 2022. https://praca.gazetaprawna.pl/artykuly/402100,minister-kopacz-ma-nowy-pomysl-na-reforme-sluzby-zdrowia.html.

———. 2010b. *Koniec z podwójnym płaceniem. W 2011 r. Kopacz wpuści na rynek prywatnych ubezpieczycieli* [No more double paying. In 2011, Kopacz will launch private insurers on the market], 20 October. Accessed 20 January 2022. https://praca.gazetaprawna.pl/artykuly/459665,koniec-z-podwojnym-placeniem-w-2011-r-kopacz-wpusci-na-rynek-prywatnych-ubezpieczycieli.html.

———. 2015. *Minister zdrowia zapowiada stopniową likwidację NFZ* [The Minister of Health announces the gradual liquidation of the National Health Fund], 1 December. Accessed 11 January 2022. https://serwisy.gazetaprawna.pl/zdrowie/artykuly/908713,radziwill-likwidacja-nfz-sluzba-zdrowia.html.

———. 2017. *Radziwiłł: likwidacja NFZ będzie, jest to kwestią czasu* [Radziwiłł: Liquidation of the National Health Fund, it is a matter of time], 1 July. Accessed 15 January 2022. https://www.gazetaprawna.pl/wiadomosci/artykuly/1054792,radziwill-likwidacja-nfz-bedzie-jest-to-kwestia-czasu.html.

Gazeta Wyborcza. 2000. Zdrowie. Prywatne kasy chorych. Spór [Health. Private health insurance. Dispute], 29 June. Accessed 12 January 2022. https://wyborcza.pl/7,75248,138949.html.

———. 2003. *Prezydent ostrzega, jakby przewidywał wyrok. NFZ niekonstytucyjny?* [The president warns, as if he is anticipating the sentence. NFZ unconstitutional?], 17 December. Accessed 12 January 2022. https://wyborcza.pl/7,75248,1830353.html.

———. 2004a. *NFZ niekonstytucyjny* [NHF unconstitutional], 7 January. Accessed 12 January 2022. https://wyborcza.pl/7,75248,1853936.html.

———. 2004b. *Po obaleniu NFZ. Kwadratura zdrowia* [After the overthrow of the National Health Fund. Health quadrature], 8 January. Accessed 12 January 2022. https://wyborcza.pl/7,75248,1855946.html.

———. 2008. *Czy Pani minister kłamie?* [Is the minister lying?], 18 June. Accessed 12 January 2022. https://wyborcza.pl/7,75968,5466556,czy-pani-minister-klamie.htm.

Golinowska, Stanisława, and Agnieszka Sowa. 2006. *Health and morbidity in the accession countries. Country report: Poland*. Brussels: European Network of Economic Policy Research Institutes, Report No. 29.

Golinowska, Stanisława, Katrazyna Tymowska, and W. Cezary Włodarczyk. 1989. *Interésie Zdrowia Społeczeństwa*. Warszawa.

Government of Poland. 1992. *Zalozenia Ogolne Ubezpieczen zdrowotnych, Miedzyresortowy Zespol do Spraw Reform zabezpieczenia Spolecznego i Systemu Swiadczen Zdrawotnych, grudzien 1992.* [General assumptions of health insurance, Interministerial Team for Social Security Reforms and Health Benefits System, December 1992.]

———. 1993. *Raport dla Pelnomocnika Rzadu d/s reformy Administracji Publicznej, przygotowal zespol pod kierunkiem J. Ruszkowskiego, Warszawa, 21 marca 1993* [Report for the Government Plenipotentiary for Public Administration Reform, prepared by a team led by J. Ruszkowski, Warsaw, March 21, 1993].

Grzymała-Busse, Anna. 2002. The programmatic turnaround of communist successor parties in East Central Europe, 1989–1998. *Communist and Post-Communist Studies* 35 (1): 51–66.

Holly, Romuald, and Magdalena Szczepaniak. 2011. The development of the private health insurance and medical services market in Poland in the years 2005–2010. *Journal of Health Policy, Insurance and Management* 1: 111–121.

Indulski, Jan, and W. Cezary Włodarczyk. 1989. *Projects of health system reform in Poland*. Paper presented at the seminar *Changing health care systems: Situation and perspective*, Kiel, 23–24 May.

Inglot, Tomasz. 2008. *Welfare States in East Central Europe, 1919–2004.* Cambridge: Cambridge University Press.

Jurkiewicz-Świętek, Irmina. 2012. Dobrowolne prywatne ubezpieczenia zdrowotne. Propozycje i debata wokół ich wprowadzenia w Polsce. *Zdrowie Publiczne i Zarządzanie* 10 (3): 156–170.

Kaasch, Alexandra. 2015. *Shaping global health policy: Global social policy actors and ideas about health care systems*. London: Palgrave Macmillan.

Kaczmarek, Krzysztof, Hannah Flynn, Edyta Letka-Paralusz, Krzysztof Krajewski-Siuda, and Christian A. Gericke. 2013. The process of privatization of health care provision in Poland. *Value in Health Regional Issues* 2 (2): 306–311.

Kaczyński, Lech. 2008. *Lech Kaczyński archive*. Office of the President of Poland. Accessed 15 January 2022. https://www.prezydent.pl/kancelaria/archiwum/archiwum-lecha-kaczynskiego/polityka-prezydenta/zdrowie-polakow.

Kaminska, Monika E., Ertila Druga, Liva Stupele, and Ante Malinar. 2021. Changing the healthcare financing paradigm: Domestic actors and international organizations in the agenda setting for diffusion of social health insurance in post-communist Central and Eastern Europe. *Social Policy & Administration* 55 (6): 1066–1081.

Karski, Jerzy B., Andrzej Koronkiewicz, and Judith Healy. 1999. *Health care systems in transition: Poland*. Copenhagen: WHO Regional Office for Europe on behalf of the European Observatory on Health Care Systems and Policies.

Klepka, Rafał. 2008. Wizje państwa w programach wyborczych z 2005 r. Platformy Obywatelskiej oraz Prawa i Sprawiedliwości. [Visions of the state in the 2005 election programs of Civic Platform and Law and Justice], Chorzowskie Studia Polityczne Wydziału Zamiejscowego w Chorzowie Wyższej Szkoły Bankowej w Poznaniu Nr 1.

Kopacz, Ewa. 2008. *Rozmawiamy z Ewa Kopacz, ministrem zdrowia* [Interview with Ewa Kopasz, Minister of Health]. *Gazeta Prawna*, 15 April. Accessed 17 January 2022. https://www.szpital.com.pl/dane/2008/aktualnosci/prasa20080415.pdf.

———. 2010. *Ewa Kopacz: Będą dodatkowe dobrowolne ubezpieczenia zdrowotne* [Ewa Kopacz: There will be additional voluntary health insurance]. Interview with E. Kopacz, 9 March. Accessed 20 January 2022. https://www.rmf24.pl/tylko-w-rmf24/wywiady/kontrwywiad/news-ewa-kopacz-beda-dodatkowe-dobrowolne-ubezpieczenia-zdrowotne,nId,241011#crp_state=1.

Krajewski-Siuda, Krzysztof, and Piotr Romaniuk. 2008. Poland—An 'experimental range' for health care system changes. Two reforms: Decentralization and centralization and their consequences. *Journal of Public Health* 16 (10): 61–70.

Kuszewski, Krzysztof, Christian Gericke, and Reiner Busse. 2005. *Health systems in transition: Poland*. Copenhagen: WHO Regional Office for Europe on behalf of the European Observatory on Health Care Systems and Policies.

Łapinski, Mariusz. 2003. *Skończył się mój czas—mówi Mariusz Łapiński, były minister zdrowia* [My time has run out—Says Mariusz Łapiński, former Minister of Health], 7 February. Accessed 15 January 2022. https://izba-lekarska.pl/numer/numer-200302/skonczyl-sie-moj-czas-mowi-mariusz-lapinski-byly-minister-zdrowia/.

Marrée, Jörgen, and Peter Groenewegen. 1997. *Back to Bismarck: Eastern European health care systems in transition*. Aldershot: Avebury.
McMenamin, Ian. 2008. Semi-presidentialism and democratization in Poland. In *Semi-presidentialism in Central and Eastern Europe*, ed. R. Elgie and S. Moestrup, 120–137. Manchester: Manchester University Press.
Mikuła, Łukasz, and Urszula Kaczmarek. 2019. From marketization to recentralization: The health-care system reforms in Poland and the post-New Public Management concept. *Revue Internationale des Sciences Administratives* 85 (1): 31–47.
Millard, L. Frances. 1982. Health care in Poland: From crisis to crisis. *International Journal of Health Services* 12 (3): 497–515.
———. 2000. Presidents and democratization in Poland: The roles of Lech Wałesa and Aleksander Kwaśniewski in building a new polity. *The Journal of Communist Studies and Transition Politics* 16 (3): 39–62.
Millard, Frances. 2003. Elections in Poland 2001: Electoral manipulation and party upheaval. *Communist and Post-Communist Studies* 36 (1): 69–86.
———. 2006. Poland's politics and the travails of transition after 2001: The 2005 elections. *Europe-Asia Studies* 58 (7): 1007–1031.
Millard, L. Frances. 2009. Poland: Parties without a party system, 1991–2008. *Politics and Policy* 37 (4): 781–798.
Ministry of Health and Social Care. 1988. *Projekt reformy systemu ochrony zdrowia i opieki społecznej. Tezy, komisja Partyjno-Rządowas Przegądu i Unowocześ niania Struktur Organizacyjnych Gospodarki i Panstwa* [Project of reform of the health protection and social welfare system. Theses, Party and Government commission for the Review and Modernization of Organizational Structures of the Economy and the State], Warszawa.
Ministry of Health and Social Welfare. 1992. *Ubespieczenia zdrawotne. Zalozenia z dnia 30 grudnia 1992, Zespol d/s Przygotowania Projektu Zalozen Ubezpieczen Zdrawotnych Komitetu Spolecznego Rady Ministrow, Warszawa* [Health insurance. Assumptions of December 30, 1992, Team for the Preparation of the Health Insurance, Social Committee of the Council of Ministers, Warsaw].
Olson, David M. 1993. Compartmentalized competition: The managed transitional election system of Poland. *The Journal of Politics* 55 (2): 415–441.
OZZL. 2022. *Saga lekarskiego protestu historia prawdziwa* [The saga of medical protest true history]. Accessed 20 May 2022. https://www.ozzl.org.pl/index.php/13890-saga-lekarskiego-protestu-historia-prawdziwa.
Pelczynski, Zbigniew, and Sergiusz Kowalski. 1990. Poland. *Electoral Studies* 9 (4): 346–354.
Pieprzyk, Paulina. 2013. The Polish health care system's endless journey to perfection: A never ending story. *Social Transformations in Contemporary Society* 1: 2345–0126.

Pilonis, Dorota. 2004. *PZ ma już rok* [Zielona Gora Agreement has a year]. *Służba Zdrowia* 9 (10): 63–66.
PiS. 2005. *Prawo i Sprawiedliwość. Program 2005: IV Rzeczpospolita—Sprawiedliwość dla wszystkich* [Law and justice. 2005 Programme: 4th Republic—Justice for all]. Accessed 15 January 2022. http://www.wybory2005.pis.org.pl/program.php.
Polish Constitutional Court. 2004. *Wyrok Trybunału Konstytucyjnego z dnia 7 stycznia 2004 r. Dz.U. nr 5 poz.37.* Accessed 20 December 2021. https://trybunal.gov.pl/postepowanie-i-orzeczenia/wyroki/art/5392-kasy-chorych-skladki-na-ubezpieczenie-zdrowotne.
Popic, Tamara. 2021a. Veto points revisited: The role of party system institutionalization in welfare state change. *Government and Opposition*: 1–22. https://doi.org/10.1017/gov.2021.37.
———. 2021b. Poland. In *Health politics in Europe: A handbook*, ed. E.M. Immergut, K.M. Anderson, C. Devitt, and T. Popic, 745–766. Oxford: Oxford University Press.
Rincker, Meg, and Martin Battle. 2011. Dissatisfied with decentralisation: Explaining citizens' evaluations of Poland's 1999 health care reforms. *Perspectives on European Politics and Society* 12 (3): 340–357.
Roberts, Andrew. 2009. The politics of healthcare reform in post-communist Europe: The importance of access. *Journal of Public Policy* 29 (3): 305–325.
Roemer, I. Milton, and Ruth Roemer. 1981. *Health care systems and comparative manpower policies.* New York: M. Dekker.
Rynek Zdrowia. 2008a. *Ewa Kopacz odkryła koszyk* [Ewa Kopacz discovered the basket], 05 June. Accessed 16 January 2022. https://www.rynekzdrowia.pl/Ubezpieczenia-zdrowotne/Ewa-Kopacz-odkryla-koszyk,323,4.html.
———. 2008b. *Wotum nieufności i plan finansowy NFZ na 2009 rok* [Vote of no confidence and NFZ financial plan for 2009], 22 July. Accessed 16 January 2022. https://www.rynekzdrowia.pl/Finanse-i-zarzadzanie/Wotum-nieufnosci-i-plan-finansowy-NFZ-na-2009-rok,751,1.html.
———. 2009. *Prezydent Lech Kaczyński podpisał ustawę o świadczeniach gwarantowanych* [President Lech Kaczyński signed the act on guaranteed benefits], 20 July. Accessed 16 January 2022. https://www.rynekzdrowia.pl/Finanse-i-zarzadzanie/Prezydent-Lech-Kaczynski-podpisal-ustawe-o-swiadczeniach-gwarantowanych,9037,1.html.
———. 2010. *Ewa Kopacz: bez ulgi podatkowej rynek polis nie ma szans* [Ewa Kopacz: The policy market has no chance without a tax relief], 6 November. Accessed 22 January 2022. https://www.rynekzdrowia.pl/Ubezpieczenia-zdrowotne/Ewa-Kopacz-bez-ulgi-podatkowej-rynek-polis-nie-ma-szans,103424,4.html.

———. 2011. *Sejm: głosowanie nad wnioskiem o odwołanie Ewy Kopacz* [Sejm: Voting on the motion to dismiss Ewa Kopacz], 26 May. Accessed 16 January 2022. https://www.rynekzdrowia.pl/Polityka-zdrowotna/Sejm-glosowanie-nad-wnioskiem-o-odwolanie-Ewy-Kopacz,109334,14.html.

Sagan, Anna, and Alicja Sobczak. 2014. Implementation of the 2011 Therapeutic Activity Act: Will commercialization improve the financial performance of Polish hospitals? *Health Policy* 118 (2): 153–158.

Sejm. 1983. *Uchwała Sejmu Polskiej Rzeczypospolitej Lodowej z dnia 29. Września 1983 r.w. sprawie ochrony zdrowia i opieki społcznej.* [Resolution of the Sejm of the Polish People's Republic of September 29, 1983 on health protection and social welfare]. Accessed 7 January 2022. https://eli.gov.pl/eli/MP/1983/175/ogl/pol.

Sitek, Michał. 2008. Politics and institutions in the reforms of health care in the Czech Republic, Hungary and Poland. *Polish Sociological Review* 161 (1): 39–53.

Słiwinski, Marian. 1980. Minister of Health speech on the Third Plenary Session of the Central Committee. *Służba Zdrowia*, July 4, 1980: 5.

Smoleń, M. Marek. 1992. The past and present of the Polish National Health Service. Reform project. *Polish Journal of Occupational Medicine and Environmental Health* 5 (1): 1–11.

Solidarity Trade Union. 1993. *Zalozenia Ubezpieczen Zdrowotnych w Polsce, Parlamentarno-Zwiazkowy Zespol Ubezpieczen Zdrowotnych NSZZ Solidarnoś ć, styczen 1993* [Foundations of health insurance in Poland, Parliamentary-Union Health Insurance Team of NSZZ Solidarność, January 1993].

Sowińska, Magda. 2010. *Zbigniew Religa walczył do końca* [Zbigniew Religa fought to the end]. Accessed 20 January 2022. https://pulsmedycyny.pl/zbigniew-religa-walczyl-do-konca-882254.

Stark, David, and Laszlo Bruszt. 1998. *Postsocialist pathways: Transforming politics and property in East Central Europe.* Cambridge: Cambridge University Press.

Szczerbiak, Aleks. 2002. Poland's unexpected political earthquake: The September 2001 parliamentary election. *The Journal of Communist Studies and Transition Politics* 18 (3): 41–76.

———. 2007. 'Social Poland' defeats 'liberal Poland'? The September–October 2005 Polish parliamentary and presidential elections. *Journal of Communist Studies and Transition Politics* 23 (2): 203–232.

Tymowska, Katarzyna. 1987. Health service financing in Poland. *The International Journal of Health Planning and Management* 2 (2): 147–157.

Włodarczyk, W. Cezary. 1987. In search of economic rationality: The experience of the Polish National Health Service. *Health Policy* 7 (2): 149–162.

Włodarczyk, W. Cezary, and Dorota Karkowska. 2000. Decentralizing the health-care sector in Poland in the 1990s. In *Decentralization in healthcare: Analyses and experiences in Central and Eastern Europe in the 1990s*, ed. George Shakarishvili. Budapest: Open Society Institute.

Włodarczyk, W. Cezary, and Piotr Mierzewski. 1991. Health services reform in Poland: Issues in recent developments. *Health Policy* 18 (1): 11–24.

World Bank. 1992. *Poland—Health system reform. A World Bank country study.* Washington, DC: The World Bank. Accessed 10 January 2022. http://documents.worldbank.org/curated/en/458211468758947430/Poland-Health-system-reform.

Żukowski, Maciej. 2013. *Country document, update 2013—Pensions, health and long-term care: Poland.* ASISP: Analytical support on social protection reforms and their socio-economic impact.

CHAPTER 6

Conclusion

Introduction

The main aim in writing this book has been to investigate the transformation of post-communist health systems, exploring *why* and *how* the trajectories of health reforms in Slovenia, Czech Republic, and Poland varied across borders and over time. The book has focused on the attempt to shift from a socialist, state-dominated health system to a system reliant on market instruments to deliver healthcare services, such as privatisation and competition. To trace the fate of the market-oriented reforms and analyse the key factors shaping them, the book combined comparative politics and public policy perspectives, emphasising that, as Gourevitch (1986) aptly put it, policy requires politics.

The definition of markets in healthcare has been discussed by academics and policymakers, with no general consensus. Therefore, the book started by conceptualising market-oriented healthcare reforms, defining them as reforms that aim to reduce the role of the state in healthcare provision (see Ewert 2009) and to influence behaviour by manipulating incentives for patients as users and doctors as producers of medical services (see Gingrich 2011). This definition distinguishes market-oriented reforms from those reforms that introduce or keep in place hierarchical 'command-and-control' systems of healthcare in which a central agency such as the state defines processes and outcomes. Thus, the book has highlighted the departure of the healthcare systems in the three countries from

T. Popic, *Health Reforms in Post-Communist Eastern Europe*,
https://doi.org/10.1007/978-3-031-15497-3_6

state-dominated, 'command-and-control' Soviet-style healthcare systems and their transformation into systems with market elements.

The book's empirical analysis has focused on three cases, selected from a larger pool of countries who pursued health reforms in the Eastern Bloc. In each of the three countries, policymakers actively sought to introduce market instruments in healthcare, but they did so with varying degrees of success, and even when they were successful, their reforms did not always stand the test of time. In Slovenia, reform efforts were marked by *survival*, as the policies introduced in the early transition stood the test of time over three decades. The Czech health policy displayed *instability*, as market elements were introduced but then partially withdrawn. Lastly, in Poland, healthcare policy showed radical *reversals* and several failed reform attempts that made the country's health system more closely resemble the previous state-dominated model. The book analysed the reform trajectories of the three countries, starting in the socialist period and concentrating on the three decades of the post-communist healthcare restructuring, from 1989 to 2019. The analysis relied on process-tracing to identify the causal processes leading to the country-specific paths and outcomes of the post-communist health reforms.

The main argument of the book is that the variation in post-communist health reforms was a result of an ideas-driven process of learning. Eastern European policymakers sought to change their healthcare systems through a series of reform initiatives that relied on market-oriented ideas and to adapt these ideas to the post-communist health policy context. However, these efforts were met with varying success because of the differences in previous experiences with markets in healthcare under socialism, institutional configurations of the new democratic states, and the patterns of political party competition.

This chapter summarises and illustrates the book's key findings. The next section compares and contrasts the three cases across the main explanatory factors: legacies, institutions and party competition. To underline how the different learning paths continue to influence policymaking, the chapter briefly compares the healthcare policy in the three countries in the context of the health crisis triggered by the COVID-19 pandemic. Lastly, it outlines the policy implications of the book's findings and concludes with a note on possible future avenues of research on healthcare reforms in Eastern Europe and beyond.

Legacies: Contrasting Slovenian, Czech, and Polish Health Reform

According to the legacy argument, previous policy regimes profoundly influence subsequent policy choices. The legacy argument has been very influential in the literature on post-socialist welfare change, supporting claims that legacies of socialism played a key role in determining post-socialist pathways (e.g. Stark and Bruszt 1998). The core argument of the book echoes this literature by saying legacies of socialism profoundly shaped post-communist policy choices. However, the book's insights go beyond the dominant views on how legacies influence policymaking. It was not the health policy legacies *per se*, but rather the experiences and perceptions of these experiences that influenced post-communist health policy choices (see Bohle and Greskovits 2012).

Slovenia had a distinctive health policy experience, as after World War II, it shifted to the Soviet-style healthcare model but kept its healthcare insurance system in place. The country's socialist regime was also the most radical in changing health policy in the context of crisis. Socialist reforms based on market ideas started in the 1970s and led to the development of a specific socialist variant of market reforms based on a unique model of organisation, 'workers' self-management'. In contrast, even though market-oriented ideas emerged in Czech and Polish health policy circles under socialism, the healthcare crisis did not catalyse significant policy change. These different responses to the socialist health crisis meant the three countries entered the post-socialist period with markedly different sets of policy experience.

These experiences influenced how the post-communist policymakers perceived the markets in healthcare. Slovenian policymakers had already experimented with alternatives to the state-led system and developed a more critical view of the role of state and market in healthcare. They knew the caveats of the state-run health system, including distortions in healthcare provision, such as shortages and corruption, but they were also aware of potential problems when provision of services is left to market-like forces, including lack of coordination, duplication of services, and rising inequalities. These critical views about the role of the state and the markets in healthcare led Slovenian post-communist reformers to take a more careful approach to market reforms. They showed an awareness of the issues that might arise in coordination and supervision of service delivery, for example, and decided not to privatise healthcare delivery. Instead, they opted to gradually introduce market elements in healthcare financing, first through patient co-payment and then by introducing complementary private health insurance.

In contrast, Czech and Polish reformers only had experience of the state-run model of healthcare provision based on central planning and the hierarchical distribution of resources. The lack of an encounter with other policy models generated indiscriminate views of alternative, market-oriented instruments for healthcare provision, feeding the perception that only radical market solutions would solve the problems of the health sector. As a result, they opted for large-scale market-oriented reforms; in both countries, these included privatisation of primary care and establishment of a managed competition model of healthcare insurance. The differences in legacies, that is, the different health policy experiences and perceptions of those experiences in post-communism explain why Slovenian policymakers were more selective, whilst Czech and Polish policymakers went for 'full' reform.

Institutions and Party Politics: Contrasting Slovenian, Czech, and Polish Health Reform

Differences in socialist legacies matter, but they cannot explain the varying paths of health reforms during the three post-communist decades. The Slovenian healthcare system kept its market elements, co-payments, and voluntary insurance, and remained unchanged throughout three decades, whilst the development of the Czech system was interrupted by frequent policy changes, and Polish health policy made a radical turn, leading to re-centralisation and resistance to subsequent marketisation attempts. The difference between the Czech and Polish health policy path is here the most striking. In both countries, initial market reforms faced implementation failures, but in the Czech case, the government regulated managed competition and continued adding other market elements, such as user fees, but in Poland, further initiatives for marketisation though private health insurance and hospital privatisation proved futile.

The book accounts for these difference by pointing to the combination of institutional veto configurations and party divisions in the context of post-communist health policymaking. The argument builds on the veto points approach but goes beyond the original view on institutional constraints (see Immergut 1992) by suggesting that looking only at institutional vetoes can be of little help in explaining stability or change in health policy. The book's argument also challenges the traditional approach to the role of partisanship in shaping policy change (see, e.g. Huber and Stephens 2001; for Eastern Europe, see Tavits and Letki 2009). In fact, the traditional left–right distinction does not capture the differential influence of party politics on post-communist health policies. Instead, to understand how political parties shaped the process of health policy learning, we need to look at the country-specific intensity of party divisions over health issues, shaped by the dynamic processes of party transformation and identity building. Taken together, the synergy of the institutional configurations and the dynamics of party politics shapes health policy.

More precisely, a combination of a light veto configuration and weak party divisions over health issues in Slovenia allowed a relatively easy retention of a country-specific model of healthcare financing strongly reliant on market elements, co-payments, and patients' complementary private healthcare insurance. The relatively weak party divisions over healthcare, characteristic of the first decade and a half of post-communism, were a result of policy agreement between the two leading parties (LDS and ZLSD/SD), one of which (ZLSD) was a successfully transformed communist successor party. The ZLSD was a successor party but wanted to make a clean break with the past and thus supported the LDS's market reforms. After the introduction of the first reforms through cross-party agreement, the combination of non-conflictual party politics and a lack of significant institutional constraints permitted a continuous and smooth learning process over time. This allowed the adaptation of market elements, such as making adjustments to the complementary private insurance (CPI), and helped handle resistance to change—two attempts to abolish the CPI and integrate it into the public health insurance scheme were unsuccessful.

In contrast, in the Czech Republic, a combination of a more constraining veto configuration and moderately intense party competition over health issues generated a context in which the learning process was protracted, making enactment of market reforms into policy more difficult. The moderate intensity of party competition was marked by a more traditional division between the right (ODS) and the social democratic left (ČSSD). The latter was a genuine social democratic party, with roots in the interwar period. As such, the party advocated left-oriented views but was also ready to move to the centre and make deals with the ODS in order to be distinguished from the other party on the left, the communist successor party (KSČM). This led to an unstable pattern of policy developments, with policy withdrawals in some cases, including user fees for services and hospital privatisation.

Lastly, in Poland, thick veto configurations, combined with intense party competition over health issues, made the adaptation of market ideas into policy particularly strenuous. The post-communist institutional design was a system with strong veto powers given to the President. The intensity of party competition was initially the result of a policy disagreement between the right-wing, post-Solidarity parties (e.g. UW, AWS) and the unreformed communist successor party (SLD), and it ultimately led to a reversal of market-oriented reform aimed at managed competition. In the context of the changed political landscape, during the second transitional decade, this conflict was replaced by a conflict between the two parties on the right (PO and PiS). Political parties' disagreements on healthcare policy goals and institutional opportunities to obstruct market reforms resulted in policy reversals and prevented the formulation of successful strategies to adapt other market reforms to the Polish health system.

Health Reforms in the Context of COVID-19

The research for this book ended in 2019, just before the outbreak of the global pandemic caused by the spread of the SARS-CoV-2 virus. The pandemic put additional pressures on healthcare systems across Europe, already strained by reduced resources and increasing demand in the context of the relatively recent global financial crisis (see Pavolini and Guillén 2013; Thomson et al. 2015; Karanikolos et al. 2013). At the same time, the spread of the virus exposed existing vulnerabilities of health systems and put under scrutiny country-specific policy choices made in the past. The most problematic policy choices were those contributing to changes in the public–private mix in health financing, reductions in hospital beds, and the creation of two-tiered healthcare systems in which access to good quality and timely care is conditional on one's ability to pay (Popic 2020; see also Johnson and Vindrola-Padros 2022).

As the pandemic swept around the world, the countries of the Eastern Bloc displayed region-specific tendencies (Popic and Moise 2021; see also Popic and Moise 2022). These countries have been praised for being exceptionally eager to introduce strict lockdown measures and hence more successfully offset the deadly effects of the pandemic for their populations compared to their Western neighbours (*The Guardian* 2020). The Eastern European countries introduced restrictive measures, such as lockdowns, early relative to the number of deaths caused by the virus (Popic and Moise 2021), but as the pandemic continued, many changed their course, relaxing the lockdowns and shifting to less restrictive measures. The effect was devastating, as some of the countries registered the world's highest COVID-19 mortality rates (*The Economist* 2020). This region's peculiar pandemic response has been explained by variety of region-specific factors, including the lack of proper democratic checks and balances,[1] thus arguably making it easier for governments to impose lockdowns (see Plümper and Neumayer 2022), but also more vulnerable health systems which rendered these countries unprepared and incapable of responding to pandemic pressures in a consistent manner (OECD 2020; see also Popic and Moise 2022).

In the context of this book, the most relevant question related to the health policy in the context of the pandemic, or more generally, the post-2019 period, is to what extent the three countries have preserved their previous policy trajectories and whether the book's argument stands the test of time. While it is still early for conclusive judgements on the effects of the pandemics on health policy in each country, it is possible to make some preliminary observations. Reports on Slovenian health policy in the post-pandemic period suggest a continuing lack of radical reforms in spite of persistent political debate surrounding the complementary private insurance, along with growing dissatisfaction of healthcare professionals (RTVSLO 2020, 2022). In the Czech Republic, health policy has been more dynamic, as shown in a recent case of a change in the elections for the boards of occupational health funds. This case reached the Constitutional Court, which ruled against the change, suggesting the judiciary is still an important veto player deciding policy battles (HSPM 2020). In Poland, the most recent reforms indicate continued efforts by the conservative (PiS) government to prevent hospital privatisation by handing hospital ownership to the State Treasury and local governments (Ministry of Health 2021). Taken together, these recent trends suggest the three countries have not changed their policy paths.

[1] Lack of democratic checks and balances refers to the tendency of some countries in the region to weaken powers of democratic institutions such as Constitutional Court, a phenomenon also referred to as 'democratic backsliding' (see Sitter and Bakke 2019).

Policy Implications

Whilst this book aims primarily at scholars and students working on the topics of health and healthcare from different disciplinary perspectives, it should also appeal to policymakers. Based on the main findings, it is possible to distinguish three relevant policy implications. One implication relates to policymakers' capacity to push for certain reforms or reform ideas, as the book's findings show this capacity is substantially shaped by the broader setting of policymaking. This setting consists of institutional structures and political dynamics embedded in the broader framework of a country's historical and political developments. To put it more succinctly, if they are willing to push for certain reform ideas, reformers will have to take account of both the structures and the agency that characterise a specific policymaking context. Settings can vary significantly in terms of institutional vetoes and political parties' willingness to support certain reforms, making it easier for reformers in some countries than in others to implement their ideas.

Another policy implication is that the barriers generated by the institutional and political settings can be overcome on some occasions, as shown in the case of the introduction of Czech user fees, passed as a fiscal measure and justified by stabilisation of the state budget. Given the fiscal pressures on governments generated by the pandemic and increased spending on health (OECD 2022), it is reasonable to expect that some of the future healthcare legislation will be justified by the need to alleviate fiscal pressures. However, as shown by the Czech example and rather than recommending opportunistic strategies, the book's findings suggest strategies that seek to overcome institutional barriers risk enacting policies contrary to the public will. They can also easily backfire and cause costly policy withdrawals.

The last policy implication relates to the role of external actors. As shown in the book, despite the lack of legislative and administrative capacity or even clear knowledge on how certain policies work in practice, the early post-communist reformers resisted foreign policy advice from actors such as the World Bank. Yet the predominantly endogenous process of post-communist health policy development has later been influenced by another external actor, the European Union. The role of the EU in health policy has been widely discussed by experts on the topic (e.g. Greer 2021), but the book's findings suggest that, as shown by the case of the Slovenian complementary health insurance, market-oriented health reforms risk going beyond the initial vision of their founders once they fall under the regulations of the EU's single market.

Future Research Agenda

As shown in this book, market-oriented reforms have been central to governments' agendas across Eastern Europe over recent decades. The book has looked mainly at what governments have done or have intended to do in terms of healthcare services and the state-market mix in providing these services to their populations. Strikingly, however, studies of post-communist public opinion show consistent and strong support for the state's role in healthcare and solidarity in healthcare provision. In the Czech Republic, for example, the share of citizens in favour of the government's role in healthcare is even higher than in European countries with strongly state-oriented welfare and healthcare systems, such as Sweden and Denmark (Missinne et al. 2013; see also Burlacu and Roescu 2021). Whilst it was beyond the scope of this book to systematically look at public opinion on healthcare and reforms, the striking support for the state's role in healthcare in face of the increasing marketisation suggests interesting avenues for future research.

References

Bohle, Dorothee, and Bela Greskovits. 2012. *Capitalist diversity on Europe's periphery*. Ithaca: Cornell University Press.

Burlacu, Diana, and Andra Roescu. 2021. Public opinion. In *Health politics in Europe: A handbook*, ed. E.M. Immergut, K.M. Anderson, C. Devitt, and T. Popic, 49–68. Oxford: Oxford University Press.

Ewert, Benjamin. 2009. Economization and marketization in the German healthcare system: How do users respond? *German Policy Studies* 5 (1): 21–44.

Gingrich, Jane. 2011. *Making markets in the welfare state: The politics of varying market reforms*. Cambridge and New York: Cambridge University Press.

Gourevitch, Peter. 1986. *Politics in hard times: Comparative responses to international economic crises*. Ithaca: Cornell University Press.

Greer, Scott L. 2021. EU health law and policy: The expansion of EU power in public health and health care. *Journal of Health Politics, Policy and Law* 46 (1): 205–210.

HSPM. 2020. Inclarity about the future of health insurance funds self-governance. Accessed 1 July 2022. https://eurohealthobservatory.who.int/monitors/health-systems-monitor/analyses/hspm/czech-republic-2015/unclarity-about-the-future-of-health-insurance-funds-self-governance.

Huber, Evelyn, and John D. Stephens. 2001. Welfare state and production regimes in the era of retrenchment. In *The new politics of the welfare state*, ed. P. Pierson, 107–145. Oxford: Oxford University Press.

Immergut, Ellen M. 1992. *Health politics: Interests and institutions in Western Europe*. Cambridge: Cambridge University Press.

Johnson, Ginger A., and Cecilia Vindrola-Padros. 2022. Lessons for current and future pandemics. In *Caring on the frontline during COVID-19*, ed. G.A. Johnson and C. Vindrola-Padros, 293–305. Singapore: Palgrave Macmillan.

Karanikolos, Marina, Philipa Mladovsky, Jonathan Cylus, Sarah J. Thomson, Sanjay Basu, David Stuckler, Johan P. Mackenbach, and Martin McKee. 2013. Financial crisis, austerity, and health in Europe. *The Lancet* 381 (9874): 1323–1331.

Ministry of Health. 2021. *Raport w sprawie zalozen reformy szpitalnictwa* [Report on the foundations of the hospital reform]. Accessed 10 July 2022. Https://www.gov.pl/web/zdrowie/raport-w-sprawie-zalozen-reformy-szpitalnictwa.

Missinne, Sarah, Bart Meuleman, and Pieter Bracke. 2013. The popular legitimacy of European healthcare systems: A multilevel analysis of 24 countries. *Journal of European Social Policy* 23: 231–247.

OECD. 2020. COVID-19 crisis response in South East European economies. Accessed 1 July 2022. Https://www.oecd.org/coronavirus/policy-responses/covid-19-crisis-response-in-south-east-european-economies-c1aacb5a/.

———. 2022. Health expenditure. Accessed 1 July 2022. Https://www.oecd.org/els/health-systems/health-expenditure.htm.

Pavolini, Emmanuele, and Anna M. Guillén. 2013. *Health care systems in Europe under austerity: Institutional reforms and performance*. Basingstoke: Palgrave Macmillan.

Plümper, Thomas, and Eric Neumayer. 2022. Lockdown policies and the dynamics of the first wave of the Sars-CoV-2 pandemic in Europe. *Journal of European Public Policy* 29 (3): 321–341.

Popic, Tamara. 2020. European health systems and COVID-19: Some early lessons. *LSE European Politics and Policy (EUROPP) Blog* (20 March 2020). Blog Entry. Accessed 12 July 2022. https://eprints.lse.ac.uk/105036/.

Popic, Tamara, and Alexandru D. Moise. 2021. *Health system resilience in the context of the COVID-19 pandemic: The gap between Eastern and Western Europe*. European University Institute. Accessed 1 July 2022. Https://www.r4rx.org/_files/ugd/6a28e0_3fe16b1b92ce437cbdc9c1d2001756d1.pdf.

———. 2022. *Government responses to the COVID-19 pandemic in Eastern and Western Europe: The role of health, political and economic factors, East European Politics*, 38(4): 507–528.

RTVSLO. 2020. *Poslanci z 51 glasovi zavrnili ukinitev dopolnilnega zdravstvenega zavarovanja* [Deputies with 51 votes rejected the abolition of supplementary health insurance]. Accessed 1 July 2022. https://www.rtvslo.si/zdravje/poslanci-z-51-glasovi-zavrnili-ukinitev-dopolnilnega-zdravstvenega-zavarovanja/512955.

———. 2022. *Težave zdravstvenega sistema se niso pojavile z epidemijo, ta jih je le še bolj razgalila.* [The problems of the health care system did not appear with the epidemic, it only exposed them even more]. Accessed 1 July 2022. https://www.rtvslo.si/slovenija/parlamentarne-volitve-2022/tezave-zdravstvenega-sistema-se-niso-pojavile-z-epidemijo-ta-jih-je-le-se-bolj-razgalila/617228.

Sitter, Nick, and Elisabeth Bakke. 2019. Democratic backsliding in the European Union. In *Oxford Research Encyclopedia of Politics.* Oxford: Oxford University Press.

Stark, David, and Laszlo Bruszt. 1998. *Postsocialist pathways: Transforming politics and property in East Central Europe.* Cambridge: Cambridge University Press.

Tavits, Margit, and Natalia Letki. 2009. When left is right: Party ideology and policy in post-communist Europe. *American Political Science Review* 103 (4): 555–569.

The Economist. 2020. Eastern Europe's Covid-19 recession could match its post-communist one. Accessed 1 July 2022. Https://www.economist.com/europe/2020/05/28/eastern-europes-covid-19-recession-could-match-its-post-communist-one.

The Guardian. 2020. Why has Eastern Europe suffered less from coronavirus than the West? Accessed 1 July 2022. Https://www.theguardian.com/world/2020/may/05/why-has-eastern-europe-suffered-less-from-coronavirus-than-the-west.

Thomson, Sarah, Josep Figueras, Tamás Evetovits, Matthew Jowett, Philipa Mladovsky, Anna Maresso, Jonathan Cylus, Marina Karanikolos, and Hans Kluge. 2015. *Economic crisis, health systems and health in Europe: Impact and implications for policy.* Copenhagen: WHO Regional Office for Europe.

Appendix: List of Interviewees

Slovenia

- Pribaković, Rade, National Institute of Public Health, 6th July 2016, Ljubljana [Interview No. 1]
- Švab, Igor, Faculty of Medicine, University of Ljubljana, 7th July 2016, Ljubljana [Interview No. 2]
- Albreht, Tit, National Institute of Public Health, 11th July 2016, Ljubljana, and e-mail correspondence [Interview No. 3]
- Stanovnik, Tine, School of Economics and Business, University of Ljubljana, 8th July 2016. [Interview No. 4]
- Bole, Velimir, Economic Institute, 7th July, 2016, Ljubljana [Interview No. 5]
- Majcen, Boris, Institute for Economic Research, University of Ljubljana, 8th July, 2016, Ljubljana [Interview No. 6]
- Kramberger, Boris, Health Insurance Institute of Slovenia, 11th July, 2016, Ljubljana [Interview No. 7]

Czech Republic

- Martin Potůček, Center for Economic Research and Graduate Education, Economics Institute, 18th September 2010 and 22nd November 2011, Prague [Interview No. 8]

T. Popic, *Health Reforms in Post-Communist Eastern Europe*,
https://doi.org/10.1007/978-3-031-15497-3

- Jaroš Jan, Czech Association for Health Service Research, 20th November 2011, Prague, and 15th December 2010, Skype interview [Interview No. 9]
- Jaroslav Volf, National Institute for Public Health, 9th November 2011, Prague [Interview No. 10]
- Petr Háva, Faculty of Social Science, Charles University, 22nd September 2010, Prague [Interview No. 11]
- Ondřej Mátl, Ministry of Health, 11th November 2011, Prague [Interview No. 12]
- Jan Richter, *Radio Prague*, 23rd September 2010, Prague [Interview No. 13]
- Martin Dlouhý, Faculty of Economics, Charles University, 9th November2011, Prague [Interview No. 14]
- Tomáš Roubal, Ministry of Health, Insurance Department, 18th September 2010, Prague [Interview No. 15]
- Tomas Machacek, Coalition for Health, 20th September 2010, Prague [Interview No. 16]
- Jan Alexa, Ministry of Health, 10th November2011, Prague [Interview No. 17]
- Schlanger Jiří, Trade Union of the Health Service and Social Care, 25th September 2010 and 18th November 2011, Prague [Interview No. 18]
- Marek Šnajdr, Deputy Minister of Health (2006–2010), 25th September 2010, Prague [Interview No. 19]

Poland

- Cezary Włodarczyk, Institute of Public Health, Jagiellonian University, 20th October 2011, Cracow [Interview No. 20]
- Piotr Romaniuk, Silesian University, Bytom, 21st October 2011, Bytom [Interview No. 21]
- Marek Góra, Warsaw School of Economics, 18th October 2011, Warsaw [Interview No. 22]
- Katarzyna Strzałkowska, Polish Chamber of Physicians, 28th September 2011, Warsaw [Interview No. 23]
- Jerzy Hausner, Faculty of Economics, 25th October 2011, Cracow [Interview No. 24]
- Krzystof Krajewski-Siuda, Institute of Public Health, Jagiellonian University, 21th October 2011, Cracow [Interview No. 25]

- Maria Swidrek, National Health Fund, Chief Specialist, 23th September 2011, Warsaw [Interview No. 26]
- Christoph Sowada, Institute of Public Health, Jagiellonian University, 21th October 2011, Cracow [Interview No. 27]
- Konstantin Radziwiłł, Polish Chamber of Physicians and Dentists, 24th October 2011, Warsaw [Interview No. 28]
- Stanislava Golinowska, Institute of Public Health, Jagiellonian University, 5th November 2011, Warsaw [Interview No. 29]
- Krzystof Bukiel, National Association of Medical Professionals, 22nd November 2011, Warsaw [Interview No. 30]

Index[1]

[1] Note: Page numbers followed by 'n' refer to notes.

T. Popic, *Health Reforms in Post-Communist Eastern Europe*,
https://doi.org/10.1007/978-3-031-15497-3

D

N

O

P

GPSR Compliance
The European Union's (EU) General Product Safety Regulation (GPSR) is a set of rules that requires consumer products to be safe and our obligations to ensure this.

If you have any concerns about our products, you can contact us on

ProductSafety@springernature.com

In case Publisher is established outside the EU, the EU authorized representative is:

Springer Nature Customer Service Center GmbH
Europaplatz 3
69115 Heidelberg, Germany

www.ingramcontent.com/pod-product-compliance
Ingram Content Group UK Ltd.
Pitfield, Milton Keynes, MK11 3LW, UK
UKHW020153290926
15471UKWH00005B/843

* 9 7 8 3 0 3 1 1 5 4 9 9 7 *